Pathology Informatics

Editor

ANIL V. PARWANI

CLINICS IN LABORATORY MEDICINE

www.labmed.theclinics.com

March 2016 • Volume 36 • Number 1

ELSEVIER

1600 John F. Kennedy Boulevard • Suite 1800 • Philadelphia, Pennsylvania, 19103-2899

http://www.theclinics.com

CLINICS IN LABORATORY MEDICINE Volume 36, Number 1
March 2016 ISSN 0272-2712, ISBN-13: 978-0-323-44408-8

Editor: Lauren Boyle
Developmental Editor: Colleen Viola

Reprints. For copies of 100 or more, of articles in this publication, please contact the Commercial Reprints Department, Elsevier Inc., 360 Park Avenue South, New York, New York 10010-1710. Tel. 212-633-3874, Fax: 212-633-3820, E-mail: reprints@elsevier.com.

Clinics in Laboratory Medicine (ISSN 0272-2712) is published quarterly by Elsevier Inc., 360 Park Avenue South, New York, NY 10010-1710. Months of issue are March, June, September, and December. Business and Editorial offices: 1600 John F. Kennedy Blvd., Suite 1800, Philadelphia, PA 19103-2899. Periodicals postage paid at NewYork, NY and additional mailing offices. Subscription prices are $250.00 per year (US individuals), $469.00 per year (US institutions), $100.00 per year (US students), $305.00 per year (Canadian individuals), $570.00 per year (Canadian institutions), $185.00 per year (Canadian students), $390.00 per year (international individuals), $570.00 per year (international institutions), $185.00 (international students). Foreign air speed delivery is included in all Clinics subscription prices. All prices are subject to change without notice. POSTMASTER: Send address changes to *Clinics in Laboratory Medicine*, Elsevier Health Sciences Division, Subscription Customer Service, 3251 Riverport Lane, Maryland Heights, MO 63043. **Customer Service: 1-800-654-2452 (US). From outside of the US and Canada, call 1-314-447-8871. Fax: 1-314-447-8029. E-mail: journalscustomerservice-usa@elsevier.com (for print support) or journalsonlinesupport-usa@elsevier.com (for online support).**

Clinics in Laboratory Medicine is covered in *EMBASE/Exerpta Medica, MEDLINE/PubMed (Index Medicus), Cinahl, Current Contents/Clinical Medicine, BIOSIS* and *ISI/BIOMED.*

Contributors

EDITOR

ANIL V. PARWANI, MD, PhD, MBA
Director of Pathology Informatics, Department of Pathology, University of Pittsburgh Medical Center, Pittsburgh, Pennsylvania

AUTHORS

DAVID R. ARTZ, MD
Medical Director, Information Systems, Memorial Sloan Kettering Cancer Center, New York, New York

KENNETH E. BLICK, PhD
Professor, Department of Pathology, University of Oklahoma Health Sciences Center, Oklahoma City, Oklahoma

DONAVAN T. CHENG, PhD
Assistant Attending, Memorial Sloan Kettering Cancer Center, New York, New York

IOAN C. CUCORANU, MD
Assistant Professor and Director of Informatics, Department of Pathology and Laboratory Medicine, University of Florida College of Medicine - Jacksonville, Jacksonville, Florida

BRYAN DANGOTT, MD
Associate Professor, Director of Pathology Informatics, East Carolina University, Greenville, North Carolina

NAVID FARAHANI, MD
Department of Pathology and Laboratory Medicine, Cedars-Sinai Medical Center, Los Angeles, California

JEFFREY L. FINE, MD
Assistant Professor; Director, Subdivision of Advanced Imaging and Image Analysis (Pathology Informatics) Department of Pathology, University of Pittsburgh School of Medicine, Pittsburgh, Pennsylvania

JIANJIONG GAO, PhD
Postdoctoral Research Fellow, Memorial Sloan Kettering Cancer Center, New York, New York

ERIC F. GLASSY, MD, FCAP
Medical Director, Affiliated Pathologists Medical Group, Torrance, California

MATTHEW G. HANNA, MD
Department of Pathology, The Mount Sinai Hospital, New York, New York

DOUGLAS J. HARTMAN, MD
Assistant Professor, Department of Anatomic Pathology, University of Pittsburgh Medical Center, Pittsburgh, Pennsylvania

LEWIS ALLEN HASSELL, MD
Professor, Department of Pathology, University of Oklahoma Health Sciences Center, Oklahoma City, Oklahoma

WALTER H. HENRICKS, MD
Medical Director, Center for Pathology Informatics; Staff Pathologist, Pathology and Laboratory Medicine Institute, Cleveland Clinic, Cleveland, Ohio

KEITH J. KAPLAN, MD
Publisher, tissuepathology.com; Pathologist and Laboratory Medical Director; Charlotte, North Carolina

LIRON PANTANOWITZ, MD
Department of Pathology, University of Pittsburgh Medical Center, Pittsburgh, Pennsylvania

B. ALAN RAMPY, DO, PhD, FCAP
Assistant Professor of Pathology, University of Texas Medical Branch, Galveston, Texas

LUIGI K.F. RAO, MD, MS
Director of Pathology Informatics and Attending Pathologist, Department of Pathology, Walter Reed National Military Medical Center, Bethesda, Maryland

SOMAK ROY, MD
Assistant Professor; Director of Genetic Services and Molecular Informatics, Department of Pathology, Molecular and Genomic Pathology, University of Pittsburgh Medical Center, Pittsburgh, Pennsylvania

NIKOLAUS SCHULTZ, PhD
Associate Attending, Memorial Sloan Kettering Cancer Center, New York, New York

S. JOSEPH SIRINTRAPUN, MD
Assistant Attending/Director of Pathology Informatics, Department of Pathology, Memorial Sloan Kettering Cancer Center, New York, New York

AIJAZUDDIN SYED, MS
Bioinformatics Engineer, Memorial Sloan Kettering Cancer Center, New York, New York

AHMET ZEHIR, PhD
Bioinformatics Engineer, Memorial Sloan Kettering Cancer Center, New York, New York

Contents

Bryan Dangott

Some laboratories or laboratory sections have unique needs that traditional anatomic and clinical pathology systems may not address. A specialized laboratory information system (LIS), which is designed to perform a limited number of functions, may perform well in areas where a traditional LIS falls short. Opportunities for specialized LISs continue to evolve with the introduction of new testing methodologies. These systems may take many forms, including stand-alone architecture, a module integrated with an existing LIS, a separate vendor-supplied module, and customized software. This article addresses the concepts underlying specialized LISs, their characteristics, and in what settings they are found.

Ioan C. Cucoranu

The main mission of a laboratory information system (LIS) is to manage workflow and deliver accurate results for clinical management. Successful selection and implementation of an anatomic pathology LIS is not complete unless it is complemented by specialized information technology support and maintenance. LIS is required to remain continuously operational with minimal or no downtime and the LIS team has to ensure that all operations are compliant with the mandated rules and regulations.

Somak Roy

Molecular informatics (MI) is an evolving discipline that will support the dynamic landscape of molecular pathology and personalized medicine. MI provides a fertile ground for development of clinical solutions to bridge the gap between clinical informatics and bioinformatics. Rapid adoption of next generation sequencing (NGS) in the clinical arena has triggered major endeavors in MI that are expected to bring a paradigm shift in the practice of pathology. This brief review presents a broad overview of various aspects of MI, particularly in the context of NGS based testing.

B. Alan Rampy and Eric F. Glassy

The underutilized practice of photographing anatomic pathology specimens from surgical pathology and autopsies is an invaluable benefit to patients, clinicians, pathologists, and students. Photographic documentation of clinical specimens is essential for the effective practice of pathology. When considering what specimens to photograph, all grossly evident pathology, absent yet expected pathologic features, and gross-only specimens should be thoroughly documented. Specimen preparation prior to photography includes proper lighting and background, wiping surfaces of blood, removing material such as tubes or bandages, orienting the specimen in a logical fashion, framing the specimen to fill the screen, positioning of probes, and using the right-sized scale.

Advanced imaging refers to direct microscopic imaging of tissue, without the need for traditional hematoxylin-eosin (H&E) microscopy, including microscope slides or whole-slide images. A detailed example is presented of optical coherence tomography (OCT), an imaging technique based on reflected light. Experience and example images are discussed in the larger context of the evolving relationship of surgical pathology to clinical patient care providers. Although these techniques are diagnostically promising, it is unlikely that they will directly supplant H&E histopathology. It is likely that OCT and related technologies will provide narrow, targeted diagnosis in a variety of in vivo (patient) and ex vivo (specimen) applications.

Telepathology is the practice of remote pathology using telecommunication links to enable the electronic transmission of digital pathology images. Telepathology can be used for remotely rendering primary diagnoses, second opinion consultations, quality assurance, education, and research purposes. The use of telepathology for clinical patient care has been limited mostly to large academic institutions. Barriers that have limited its widespread use include prohibitive costs, legal and regulatory issues, technologic drawbacks, resistance from pathologists, and above all a lack of universal standards. This article provides an overview of telepathology technology and applications.

The single most important element to consider when evaluating clinical information systems for a practice is workflow. Workflow can be broadly defined as an orchestrated and repeatable pattern of business activity enabled by the systematic organization of resources into processes that transform materials, provide services, or process information.

This article provides surgical pathologists an overview of health information systems (HISs): what they are, what they do, and how such systems relate to the practice of surgical pathology. Much of this article is dedicated to the electronic medical record. Information, in how it is captured, transmitted, and conveyed, drives the effectiveness of such electronic medical record functionalities. So critical is information from pathology in integrated clinical care that surgical pathologists are becoming gatekeepers of not only tissue but also information. Better understanding of HISs can empower surgical pathologists to become stakeholders who have an impact on the future direction of quality integrated clinical care.

Translational bioinformatics and clinical research (biomedical) informatics
are the primary domains related to informatics activities that support translational research. Translational bioinformatics focuses on computational
techniques in genetics, molecular biology, and systems biology. Clinical
research (biomedical) informatics involves the use of informatics in discovery and management of new knowledge relating to health and disease.
This article details 3 projects that are hybrid applications of translational
bioinformatics and clinical research (biomedical) informatics: The Cancer
Genome Atlas, the cBioPortal for Cancer Genomics, and the Memorial
Sloan Kettering Cancer Center clinical variants and results database, all
designed to facilitate insights into cancer biology and clinical/therapeutic
correlations.

This article presents an overview of the curriculum deemed essential for
trainees in pathology, with mapping to the Milestones competency statements. The means by which these competencies desired for pathology
graduates, and ultimately practitioners, can best be achieved is discussed.
The value of case (problem)-based learning in this realm, in particular the
kind of integrative experience associated with hands-on projects, to both
cement knowledge gained in the lecture hall or online and to expand competency is emphasized.

CLINICS IN LABORATORY MEDICINE

THE CLINICS ARE NOW AVAILABLE ONLINE!
Access your subscription at:
www.theclinics.com

Laboratory Information Systems

Walter H. Henricks, MD

KEYWORDS

- Laboratory information systems • Informatics • Laboratory operations
- Laboratory management • Computer systems • Pathology informatics • Workflow

OVERVIEW TO LABORATORY INFORMATION SYSTEMS

Pathologists and pathology laboratories depend on laboratory information systems (LISs) to support their operations and, ultimately, to carry out their patient care mission. Over the past few decades,[1,2] LISs have evolved from relatively narrow, often arcane, and/or home-grown systems into sophisticated systems that are more user-friendly and support a broader range of functions and integration with other technologies that laboratories deploy.

Modern LISs consist of complex, interrelated computer programs and infrastructure that support a vast array of information-processing needs of laboratories. LISs have functions in all phases of patient testing, including specimen and test order intake, specimen processing and tracking, support of analysis and interpretation, and report creation and distribution. In addition, LISs provide management reports and other data that laboratories need to run their operations and to support continuous improvement and quality initiatives.

This article describes the structure and functions of anatomic pathology LISs (APLISs), with emphasis on their roles in laboratory operations and their relevance to pathologists.

ELEMENTS OF LABORATORY INFORMATION SYSTEMS
Laboratory Information System Infrastructure

LISs have a foundation of technical infrastructure. Such infrastructure consists in aggregate of hardware and related dedicated software that enable the LIS to carry out its functions (**Box 1**). Software is computer programming that consists of instructions for the components of the computer system to perform.

This article originally appeared in Surgical Pathology Clinics, Volume 8, Issue 2, June 2015.
The author has no competing financial interests to disclose.
Center for Pathology Informatics, Pathology and Laboratory Medicine Institute, Cleveland Clinic, L21, 9500 Euclid Avenue, Cleveland, OH 44195, USA
E-mail address: henricw@ccf.org

> **Box 1**
> **Laboratory information system (LIS) infrastructure components**
>
> - Servers
> - End-user devices: desktop PCs
> - Monitors
> - Printers: paper and label
> - Scanners
> - Networks

Servers are computers that house the main elements of the LIS software, including its main database (see later in this article). Servers provide, or "serve," LIS functions to system users and/or other processes (eg, printers) that request them. Servers can accommodate simultaneous access by multiple users in a networked system environment. An LIS may use one or more servers, and some servers may be dedicated to specific functions like managing communications with other systems (ie, interfaces).

LIS users (sometimes referred to as "end-users") in the laboratory gain access to the LIS through end-user devices, most commonly desktop computers (in this article generically referred to as PCs for personal computer). In a client-server environment (see later in this article), these devices are referred to as *client* devices. Use of LISs on other client devices, such as tablets and smartphones, is emerging as well.[3,4]

LISs require the use of networking technologies for connections among the LIS infrastructure components. Networks consist of physical media and related engineering software that together enable electronic data exchange. Networks in an LIS may include copper (Ethernet), fiber optics, wireless, and/or other media. The network to which an LIS is connected within an organization typically can gain access to the worldwide network of the Internet by way of an organization's gateway to external networks.

LISs also connect to various peripheral devices to execute certain functions. Computer display monitors are an obvious requirement at an end-user PC. The specification requirements for display monitors are getting increasing attention with the advent of whole slide imaging techniques and virtual microscopy, that bring with them need for higher-resolution displays.[5] Printers are necessary for printing reports, and label printers of different form factors print labels for slides, specimen containers, and other assets. Digital scanners enable the capture of hard copy elements, such as paper requisitions or insurance information, into an LIS.

Laboratory Information System Architecture

LIS architecture affects users' LIS experience. The *architecture* of an LIS refers to the model of how the hardware and software components function together to deliver LIS functions. LIS architecture defines the allocation of computing power among system components. LISs are commonly deployed as some variant of *client-server* architecture (**Fig. 1**). In client-server, end-users invoke LIS functions on their "client" devices. The functions go to servers as requests for services, for example editing a report, electronic sign out, data entry, or accessioning a case. Clients and servers work together to perform system functions, and computing resources and power are "distributed" in this manner.

Although older, the *mainframe*, or host-based, architecture exists in some LISs (**Fig. 2**). Mainframe set ups differ from client-server in that computing resources are

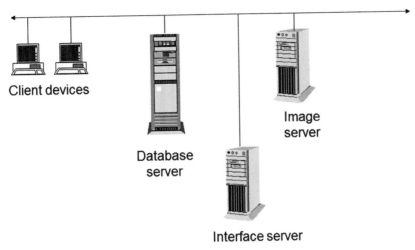

Fig. 1. Client-server LIS architecture.

centralized to a much greater degree on a single powerful computer ("mainframe"). The mainframe, or host, manages all LIS functions. Instead of using computing devices with software, end-users interact with the system using so-called "dumb" terminals that function only for data input and display functions.

Many laboratories now benefit from use of *thin client* LIS architecture (**Fig. 3**). In the thin client model, LIS client software is centralized onto a thin client-server, and end-users interact with the LIS by using client software that performs only simple functions (= "thin" client) for communicating with the thin client-server. The benefits for laboratories of using thin client in an LIS are listed in **Box 2**. In short, thin client architecture greatly facilitates system administration by standardizing the client software available to users and because client software updates need only occur on the thin client-server(s) instead of on all individual PCs. Laboratories should be aware, however, that using thin client may incur additional license costs, and not all LIS functions may be available to users who access the LIS via thin client. For example,

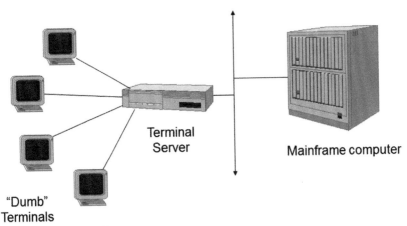

Fig. 2. Mainframe LIS architecture.

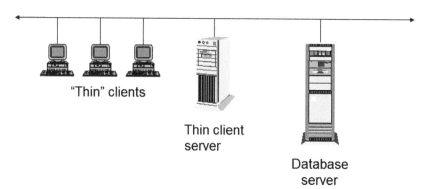

"Thin" clients

Thin client
server

Database
server

Fig. 3. Thin client LIS architecture.

speech-to-text recognition or digital image capture into the LIS may not be possible using a thin client to access the system.

In what can be thought of as an extension of the thin client model, hospitals and laboratories are increasingly choosing to implement LISs based on software-as-a-service (SaaS) arrangement with an LIS vendor. These models are also referred to application service provider and "in the cloud." In these settings, a laboratory contracts with a vendor to provide an LIS application over secure network or Internet connections with the system that the vendor maintains at a remote location. An SaaS arrangement offers laboratories benefits that include a lower cost of acquisition and the outsourcing of infrastructure and software maintenance and upgrades. On the other hand, the laboratory is reliant on the vendor to maintain high availability of the system, and the options for configuration or customization of LIS functions may be limited.

THE HEART OF AN LABORATORY INFORMATION SYSTEM: DICTIONARY TABLES AND DEFINITIONS

An LIS is at its core a database, and data are typically organized into tables or files that relate to one another based on system logic. Databases are described in detail in the article by Parwani elsewhere in this issue. Operating within the LIS, a database management system controls the access, organization, storage, management, retrieval, and integrity of data that reside in the LIS database. Broadly speaking, LIS tables are of 2 types: *record tables* and *maintenance tables*. Record tables consist of data generated during the course of using the system for patient care activities, ranging from daily logs to long-term archive of pathology reports. Maintenance tables define

---

Box 2
Benefits of thin client LIS

- Easier administration
- Central control and standardization of LIS software
- LIS software updates
- Leveraging of legacy desktop hardware: prolonged useful life
- Support of multiple device types in same environment
- User access to LIS from off-site locations (remote access)

and keep track of information about the system is configured, including data definitions and internal system operations.

LIS *dictionaries* are the maintenance tables in the LIS that determine and store the data definitions, terminology, naming conventions, report content and format, and other configurations for the laboratory. These definitions ultimately determine workflow and processes in the laboratory. The typical LIS contains dozens of dictionaries. Examples of important dictionaries in an APLIS are listed in **Box 3**.

LIS dictionary definitions tailor the LIS to the unique needs and expectations of an individual laboratory. Definition building requires planning, allocation of resources, and understanding of the laboratory's desired operations. Careful attention to establishing table definitions in the LIS is crucial to successful LIS implementation and smooth operations. Although an LIS may have some "out-of-the-box" default table entries, the laboratory will need to review default entries carefully to determine acceptability.

Change control processes for LIS dictionaries merit consideration. When a laboratory desires to make changes to LIS definitions, even seemingly minor changes can lead to unintended and/or negative consequences. For example, when a laboratory discontinues use of a particular special stain, if dictionary entries are not properly updated, the stain code may remain embedded in some histology stain-ordering protocols and appear to be requested of the laboratory. This example also illustrates the important point that some dictionary entries are linked to entries in other tables or definitions and that knowledge of these relationships is important in managing changes.

FEATURES OF ANATOMIC PATHOLOGY LABORATORY INFORMATION SYSTEMS AND THEIR ROLES IN LABORATORY OPERATIONS

The APLIS has numerous "touch points" in pathology laboratory workflow throughout the specimen analysis and interpretation cycle. The following subsections describe roles of the LIS functions and data elements in preanalytic, analytical, and postanalytic phases of testing in the surgical pathology laboratory. Generally, these processes correspond to functional modules in the LIS that link to one another.

Specimen Intake and Accessioning

On receipt of a specimen in the laboratory, the first step in processing is to register, or to "accession" the specimen into the LIS. This is the point at which the LIS first "learns"

Box 3
Anatomic pathology LIS (APLIS) example dictionaries

- Security/access level privileges for user classes (eg, technologist vs pathologist)
- Pathologist names and data
- Clinician names and data
- Patient locations
- Laboratory areas
- Specimen categories (eg, cytology, surgical pathology)
- Specimen types (eg, colon resection, prostate biopsy)
- Histology stain protocols
- Text templates ("boilerplate")
- Fee codes and billing rules

of the existence of the new specimen. Laboratory personnel enter patient-specific and specimen-specific data that are present on a requisition that accompanies the specimen; such requisitions (or test request forms, or "req's") are typically hard copy (in anatomic pathology), although electronic transmission of anatomic pathology orders from an electronic health record (EHR) to the LIS are possible.[6]

Correct patient-specimen identification is of paramount importance when accessioning. In health care institutional settings, the APLIS typically receives a regular electronic feed of patient demographic information via an interface with the institution's patient registration/management system. These "ADT" (admission-discharge-transfer) interfaces supply the LIS with data that (depending on the circumstances) include patient names, medical record numbers, gender, data of birth, location, physician, insurance, and others. An ADT feed enables laboratory users to select and to pull into the LIS all the necessary demographic data after entering only a name or medical record number. This process reduces the risk of patient misidentification or selection of the incorrect patient. In settings without an ADT feed to the LIS, new patient demographic records must be created in the LIS for patients not seen previously.

The other data elements entered during accessioning are typically a mixture of free-text entries and selection from dictionary entries defined for a particular data field. For example, the user will select a submitting physician from choices displayed from entries defined in the LIS Physician Dictionary. Other data elements that are commonly captured at accessioning are listed in **Box 4**. Additionally, dictionary elements, such as orders for histology protocols and default fee codes, can attach to the case (or part) automatically based on rules and linkages to specimen types that the laboratory defines in the LIS.

The outcome of the accessioning process is the LIS assigning a unique LIS accession number (case number) to the case. The LIS updates the specimen status to "accessioned" (or something analogous). Accession numbers are typically a combination of letters and numbers, and a laboratory may define various "number wheels" in the LIS to distinguish different categories of specimens (eg, by originating location,

---

Box 4
Data elements entered into APLIS at time of case accessioning

- Patient identification number
- Patient name and other identifying information
- Specimen type[a] (eg, colon biopsy)
- Specimen description (eg, mass in gastric body)
- Submitting physician[a]
- "Copy to" physician(s)[a]
- Patient location[a] and/or client location[a]
- Date of procedure
- Date of receipt
- Pathologist assigned[a]
- Clinical history
- Histology protocols linked to specimen type[a]

[a] Indicates that entry is selected based on LIS dictionary entries.

HS-15-123, CS-15-123). The LIS assigns a single accession number to cases that have multiple individual specimen parts (eg, multiple prostate needle biopsies). This capability keeps the case cohesive and enables a single report for multispecimen cases. By contrast, clinical laboratory LISs typically assign a unique number to each individual specimen container (eg, blood tubes), and a separate result is provided for multiple tests ordered on the specimen.

Gross Specimen Processing and Sectioning ("Grossing")

The gross processing phase begins with generation of a gross description of the specimen and ends with submission and designation of sections for histologic slide preparation. Users enter gross descriptions into the gross description field in the LIS. Defining specimen type-specific boilerplate, template text entries in LIS dictionaries can facilitate text entry. Many LISs also incorporate or accommodate speech-to-text ("voice recognition") entry, which can reduce reliance on transcription and speed processing.[7] Sections selected for histology designated in the gross description follow the laboratory-defined numbering scheme in the LIS for specimen parts and tissue blocks (eg, A1, A2, B1, B2). At the completion of sectioning, the prosector or other processor creates discrete entries in the designated tissue sections/blocks in the histology module (or similar), in preparation for the next steps. At the end of the grossing process and entries, the case status in the LIS can be updated to "Gross Complete," or something similar.

To optimize specimen identification and *specimen tracking*, a pathology laboratory may deploy an electronic interface between the LIS and cassette engravers that label the cassettes into which prosectors place tissue sections. Such interfaces establish a link between the asset (tissue cassette/block) and the LIS to improve specimen identification and tracking.[8] Data engraved on cassettes may include bar codes, particularly 2-dimensional bar codes, which increase data available to the LIS and other systems compatible with the bar code(s). Radiofrequency identification technologies hold promise as a future method for asset tracking once barriers of cost and system integration have been overcome.[9,10]

Histology Processing and Slide Creation

Histology laboratory processing begins with tissue fixation and preparation of tissue blocks and ends with creation of glass slides with stained tissue sections. Throughout this phase of processing, the LIS tracks and organizes the workflow in the laboratory, largely through the use of histology logs and histology protocols. The LIS logs are essentially lists of the specimens that a particular bench or area of the laboratory will process for an upcoming specified period of time (eg, work shift). The specimen data on the logs corresponds to data entered "upstream," for instance the tissue cassettes designated as submitted in the grossing phase. LIS histology logs often in use include embedding logs, routine histology logs, special stain request logs, and immunohistochemistry logs. A laboratory can configure the format of the logs and the data to be displayed, or may choose the system's default configurations. Data elements in histology logs typically include accession number, date/time stamp, patient and specimen data, histology protocol(s) ordered, other stains ordered, and comments about the specimen or the request.

Histology protocols are LIS dictionary entries that define the number of slides/levels, histologic stains, and other instructions for processing. For routine workflow (particularly for biopsies), these protocols often attach to the specimen part automatically during the accessioning process (see earlier in this article) and appear on logs that the LIS automatically prints at laboratory-defined intervals. For add-on stains, users order stains, protocols, or batteries of stains in the LIS by selecting from dictionary entries provided in the stain-ordering function. These protocol orders then appear on the corresponding log for the laboratory.

An LIS may support individual slide tracking.[8] At microtomy stations, a laboratory may deploy a combination of barcode scanners and slide labelers/engravers to enable histotechnologists to track each block and slide and to ensure concordance of identification between individual block and slide labels. These functions depend on connections with the LIS for data exchange and comparisons. LISs typically offer at least some capability for the laboratory to determine the format and content of its slide labels.

Pathologist Interpretation and Final Report Generation and Distribution

For each case, a "working draft" report in the LIS provides the pathologist with information about the case and processing up to the point that he or she has received the slides. The laboratory may choose to provide hard copies of working drafts, printed in batch mode and collated with the slides for each case, or pathologists may access working drafts paperlessly in the LIS. The laboratory can configure the format and content of working drafts in the LIS. Working drafts typically include gross description, including sections submitted, clinical information, frozen section results (as applicable), default fee codes, and data about the patient's previous pathology specimens available in the LIS.

Pathologists, or designees such as transcriptionists, enter pathologic diagnosis and, as applicable, descriptive comments and microscopic description, into the relevant data fields in the LIS. To facilitate entry of diagnosis text, an LIS may include capabilities such as speech-to-text conversion ("voice recognition")[7,11,12] and creation of predefined templates, checklists, and formats. Default codes for billing (Current Procedural Terminology) and/or diagnosis (International Classification of Diseases) codes linked to specimen type definitions may auto-populate into final reports.

Final diagnosis data fields in LISs are typically entered and stored as text "blobs" that are not further structured in the database. Even if a report template enables display of report content in a structured manner (eg, as a checklist or "synoptic" report), such display alone does not correspond to structure with discrete data elements in the underlying database. Some LISs and third-party solutions offer so-called true "synoptic" modules that enable report data entry and storage as discrete data elements,[13,14] which are then amenable to more effective criteria-based database query and analysis. Synoptic reporting is covered more extensively in the article by Parwani elsewhere in this issue.

Once a report is finalized, the LIS supports distribution of the reports, whether electronic or hard copy. A pathologist finalizes a report (ie, "signs out" a case) by entering an electronic signature (or by otherwise marking it as final if manual signatures are used), which locks the case in the database. For certain types of reports, or for certain physician groups, a laboratory may need to fax or to print remotely hard copies, and the LIS sends these reports based on rules and definitions (eg, recipient fax number). If there is an LIS-EHR interface for results, finalizing a report triggers transmission of the report to the EHR.

In EHRs, the screen design and formatting dictates the quality and readability of the display of interfaced pathology reports. Sometimes reports may appear quite different in the EHR compared with the LIS, with potential for misinterpretation.[15,16] An LIS may be able to provide interfaced electronic reports that preserve formatting (eg, portable document format, PDF), and if the receiving system can accommodate such reports, this may be a mechanism for improving readability.

Report Amendments and Addenda

LISs accommodate amended reports and report addenda through similar though not identical ways. Once an electronic signature is affixed to a report in the LIS, the report cannot be changed without creating an amendment, or amended report. If a report is changed or corrected, the LIS automatically marks the amended case as such in the database and automatically labels any new reports generated from the case as amended reports. An LIS may have the capability to categorize and to display the reasons for the amendment. An addendum report is created in the LIS in cases when new information, such as special stain results, is added to a previously finalized report. Addenda do not involve changing any information in the original report. Pathologists finalize amended and addended reports with a new electronic signature.

In the setting of an LIS-EHR interface, the amended report replaces and overlays the original report in the EHR. The same may be true for addenda, but depending on the setting, addenda may be appended to cases without completely overlaying the previous. Laboratories may have to ensure that amended or addended status is obvious in the format and display of reports in the LIS and the EHR. Audit trail functions ensure that original reports are accessible in the LIS and the EHR.

The Laboratory Information System and Laboratory Administration

In addition to the capabilities necessary for daily operations and patient care in the laboratory, the LIS offers functions that support management and leadership activities in the laboratory. Laboratories rely on *management reports* from the LIS for data that reflect status of operations, laboratory performance, metrics, and maintenance. **Box 5** lists common categories of management reports in an APLIS. Laboratories will typically have options of using management reports that are predefined in the LIS, modifying predefined reports, or creating their own LIS management reports. LISs accommodate scheduling of management reports to fire off automatically at defined times or intervals (eg, every morning), and laboratory personnel can run reports on an ad hoc basis.

LISs provide for quality management activities beyond management reports. A laboratory may be able to configure its LIS to select cases automatically and randomly for secondary quality assurance review and assign to a second pathologist.[17] In residency training programs, LISs can track aspects of resident performance. Gynecologic cytopathology has multiple quality and regulatory requirements that LISs often have tools to facilitate.

LISs have tools for database queries. Although management reports are a type of database query, laboratories often need to conduct database searches based on criteria tailored to a specific question or need. Common examples are case finding

---

Box 5
Categories of common management reports in an APLIS

- Turnaround time (TAT)
- Cases not signed out (ie, pending case logs)
- Volumes of specimens, blocks, slides
- Utilization (eg, special stains)
- Billing reports
- Interface error logs

for validation or development of stains in the laboratory, quality reviews, and investigative research. Efficacy of database searches in an LIS depends on the structure of underlying data (ie, discrete data elements vs unstructured text) and on the LIS tools available to define queries. More on database structures and data elements can be found in the articles by Parwani and Amin elsewhere in this issue.

ADVANCED FEATURES AND FUNCTIONS IN LABORATORY INFORMATION SYSTEMS

LISs now incorporate multiple features that were either unavailable or that not long ago required custom development.[18] Recently, the Association for Pathology Informatics created and published a detailed listing of basic and advanced LIS features as part of a toolkit to assess LIS capabilities.[19] Several such capabilities (speech-to-text conversion ["voice recognition"], barcoding, specimen/block/slide tracking, engraver interfaces) have been described in their context of laboratory operations in earlier sections of this article. LISs now routinely possess capabilities to store digital images linked to cases. With the increasing acceptance of whole slide imaging (WSI) for clinical purposes,[20,21] capabilities for interfaces or integration between WSI systems and LIS will likely increase. Various aspects of imaging in pathology are covered in other articles of this text.

With respect to further advances, future LISs are expected to have more sophisticated tools to support data mining and pathologists' analysis of pathology and clinical data sets.[22] Some experts believe that the LIS will evolve into multimodality pathologist "cockpits" that combine pathology imaging, access to clinical data (eg, EHR) and other data sources, LIS functions, and analytical tools.[23] As applications for molecular genetic pathology testing, including next generation sequencing, on pathology specimens continue to emerge, further innovation in LISs will be necessary to report and to correlate such data in concert with traditional pathologic findings in ways that are optimal for patient care.[24]

REFERENCES

1. Elevitch FR, Aller RD. The ABCs of LIS: computerizing your laboratory information system. Chicago: ASCP Press; 1989.
2. Carter AB, McKnight RM, Henricks WH, et al. Pathology informatics: an introduction. In: Pantanowitz L, Tuthill JM, Balis UJ, editors. Pathology informatics: theory and practice. Chicago: ASCP Press; 2012. p. 1–10.
3. Park S, Parwani A, Satyanarayanan M, et al. Handheld computing in pathology. J Pathol Inform 2012;3:15.
4. Hartman DJ, Parwani AV, Cable B, et al. Pocket pathologist: a mobile application for rapid diagnostic surgical pathology consultation. J Pathol Inform 2014;5:10.
5. Krupinski EA. Virtual slide telepathology workstation of the future: lessons learned from teleradiology. Hum Pathol 2009;40(8):1100–11.
6. Georgiou A, Westbrook J, Braithwaite J. Computerized provider order entry systems: research imperatives and organizational challenges facing pathology services. J Pathol Inform 2010;1:11.
7. Henricks WH, Roumina K, Skilton BE, et al. The utility and cost effectiveness of voice recognition technology in surgical pathology. Mod Pathol 2002;15(5):565–71.
8. Pantanowitz L, Mackinnon AC Jr, Sinard JH. Tracking in anatomic pathology. Arch Pathol Lab Med 2013;137(12):1798–810.
9. Leung AA, Lou JJ, Mareninov S, et al. Tolerance testing of passive radio frequency identification tags for solvent, temperature, and pressure conditions

encountered in an anatomic pathology or biorepository setting. J Pathol Inform 2010;1:21.

10. Bostwick DG. Radiofrequency identification specimen tracking in anatomical pathology: pilot study of 1067 consecutive prostate biopsies. Ann Diagn Pathol 2013;17(5):391–402.

11. Kang HP, Sirintrapun SJ, Nestler RJ, et al. Experience with voice recognition in surgical pathology at a large academic multi-institutional center. Am J Clin Pathol 2010;133(1):156–9.

12. Singh M, Pal TR. Voice recognition technology implementation in surgical pathology: advantages and limitations. Arch Pathol Lab Med 2011;135(11):1476–81.

13. Kang HP, Devine LJ, Piccoli AL, et al. Usefulness of a synoptic data tool for reporting of head and neck neoplasms based on the College of American Pathologists cancer checklists. Am J Clin Pathol 2009;132(4):521–30.

14. Hassell LA, Parwani AV, Weiss L, et al. Challenges and opportunities in the adoption of College of American Pathologists checklists in electronic format: perspectives and experience of Reporting Pathology Protocols Project (RPP2) participant laboratories. Arch Pathol Lab Med 2010;134(8):1152–9.

15. Valenstein PN. Formatting pathology reports: applying four design principles to improve communication and patient safety. Arch Pathol Lab Med 2008;132(1):84–94.

16. Wilkerson ML, Henricks WH, Castellani WJ, et al. Management of laboratory information in the electronic health record. Arch Pathol Lab Med 2015;139(3):319–27.

17. Owens SR, Dhir R, Yousem SA, et al. The development and testing of a laboratory information system-driven tool for pre-sign-out quality assurance of random surgical pathology reports. Am J Clin Pathol 2010;133(6):836–41.

18. Sinard JH, Gershkovich P. Custom software development for use in a clinical laboratory. J Pathol Inform 2012;3:44.

19. Tuthill JM, Friedman BA, Balis UJ, et al. The laboratory information system functionality assessment tool: ensuring optimal software support for your laboratory. J Pathol Inform 2014;5:7.

20. Pantanowitz L, Sinard JH, Henricks WH, et al, College of American Pathologists Pathology and Laboratory Quality Center. Validating whole slide imaging for diagnostic purposes in pathology: guideline from the College of American Pathologists Pathology and Laboratory Quality Center. Arch Pathol Lab Med 2013;137(12):1710–22.

21. Bauer TW, Schoenfield L, Slaw RJ, et al. Validation of whole slide imaging for primary diagnosis in surgical pathology. Arch Pathol Lab Med 2013;137(4):518–24.

22. Sepulveda JL, Young DS. The ideal laboratory information system. Arch Pathol Lab Med 2013;137(8):1129–40.

23. Krupinski EA. Optimizing the pathology workstation "cockpit": challenges and solutions. J Pathol Inform 2010;1:19.

24. Gu J, Taylor CR. Practicing pathology in the era of big data and personalized medicine. Appl Immunohistochem Mol Morphol 2014;22(1):1–9.

Bar Coding and Tracking in Pathology

Matthew G. Hanna, MD[a],*, Liron Pantanowitz, MD[b]

KEYWORDS

- Bar codes • Tracking • Pathology informatics • RFID

OVERVIEW

Bar codes are standardized identification tools that allow for asset tracking. They have widespread use in point of sale purchases, delivery companies, automobile industry, and health care. With advances in technology over the past few decades, there have been tremendous improvements in bar code and scanner performance. Some of the main purposes of implementing a bar coding and tracking system are to reduce errors and increase efficiency. Instead of manual logging entries, bar coding has reduced human errors by automating identification and tracking. Regarding health care, bar coding is a hospital-wide operation. From patient wristbands to hospital beds, different bar codes or RFID tags are used to identify, locate, and audit labeled assets.

The clinical laboratory has demonstrated positive effects of implementing bar coding and tracking systems.[1–6] Similar use of this technology, however, has only recently been introduced in anatomic pathology. Ever-increasing specimen volumes, complex testing, and a desire for decreased turnaround times without increasing costs and errors provide a pressing impetus for pathology laboratories to implement tracking solutions. There are myriad pathology assets that can be identified and tracked, including order requisitions, specimen containers, tissue cassettes/blocks, glass slides, and reagents. Interfacing bar codes or RFID tags with the LIS have become essential for contemporary pathology laboratories to reap the benefits of asset tracking, such as driving workflow, automation, error reduction, digital pathology, and improved patient safety.

HISTORY

Bar codes, which are ubiquitous today, made their debut approximately 80 years ago (**Table 1**). The first mention of bar coding was US patent 1985035A, published on

This article originally appeared in Surgical Pathology Clinics, Volume 8, Issue 2, June 2015.
Disclosure Statement: The authors have no disclosures.
[a] Department of Pathology, The Mount Sinai Hospital, 1 Gustave L Levy Place, New York, NY 10029, USA; [b] Department of Pathology, University of Pittsburgh Medical Center, 5150 Centre Avenue, Pittsburgh, PA 15232, USA
* Corresponding author.
E-mail address: matthew.hanna@mountsinai.org

Table 1 Historical events of bar codes	
Date	**Event**
December 18, 1934	US patent 1985035A is the first mention of bar code technology
October 20, 1949	US Patent 2612994A filed, describes the first bar code process
1961	Color bar codes first used on railroad cars
June 23, 1973	Announcement of the first UPC point of sale system
June 26, 1974	First product bar code scanned in a supermarket (Wrigley gum)
September 21, 1981	US Department of Defense adopts Code 39 bar code
September 1982	US Postal Service use POSTNET bar code to represent zip codes
1987	ISO 9000 quality management standards first created
February 2004	US Food and Drug Administration requires medications use bar codes
October 12, 2005	AABB requires ISBT 128 bar code for accreditation

Abbreviations: AABB, American Association of Blood Banks; POSTNET, Postal Numeric Encoding Technique.
Adapted from UPC History. ID History Museum.[7]

December 18, 1934, by John Kermode, Douglass Young, and Harry Sparkes. Their patent included "sorting machines which employ photo-electric cells or other light-responsive means for sorting cards, records or the like in response to a code or designation marked thereon, or for tabulating, recording or effecting other controls in accordance with the marks on the cards or records." In October 1949, Norman Woodland and Silver Bernard filed a patent (US patent 2612994A), which delineated the first bar code process, entitled "Classifying apparatus and method." Bernard and Woodland were devising a method to automatically scan products at grocery stores to minimize time in checkout lines. Woodland eventually continued developing bar codes at IBM. The earliest bar coding system was used in a railroad company to identify railroad cars, called KarTrak automatic car identification. This color bar code system has many similarities to bar codes in use today. KarTrak used 13 horizontal labels of different width and spacing, a start and stop line, and a line checker. Due to high human reading error rates, however, their system was abandoned in the 1970s. The supermarket industry started using candidate bar code formats for automated checkout systems in the mid-1960s. In 1973, after many ad hoc committee meetings, the uniform product code (UPC) was designated the national standard by the National Association of Food Chains for grocery product identification. The International Organization for Standardization (ISO) 9000 quality-management standards, first created in 1987, have pushed companies to ensure compliance with bar coding systems.[7–9] Because of these advancements, bar codes have a global presence. Health care subsequently also widely adopted bar code technology.

TYPES OF BAR CODES

A bar code is defined as an optical machine-readable symbol representing a set of data. Bar codes use light reflection on different-sized white and black bars or dots to encode a binary (1s and 0s) string of data. There are hundreds of different bar code varieties that can be created, most of which are grouped into categories of a linear (1-D) or 2-D bar code symbology (**Fig. 1**). The mapping between the bar code and message is called a symbology. Bar code symbology defines the technical details of a particular type of bar code (eg, encodable character set, bar spacing and width,

Fig. 1. Linear (1-D) and 2-D bar code symbology examples. 1-D bar codes with data encoded only on the horizontal axis are represented by differentially spaced and sized line bars. 2-D symbologies are represented as black and white dots with data encoded along the vertical and horizontal axis.

and checksum specifications). 1-D symbologies include numeric or alphanumeric data. 2-D symbologies can include a much greater character count (higher data density), require a smaller footprint, and have fewer scan and printer failures compared with 1-D symbologies.[10–12] There is no single bar code that encompasses all uses and needs of a laboratory; consequently, using a combination of symbologies is commonplace and recommended based on a particular laboratory's needs. In efforts to standardize bar coding in laboratories, the Clinical and Laboratory Standards Institute (CLSI) published AUTO02-A2 (Laboratory Automation: Bar Codes for Specimen Container Identification) and AUTO12-A (Specimen Labels: Content and Location, Fonts, and Label Orientation).[13,14] These guidelines established an April 29, 2014, deadline for laboratories to comply with bar code standardization on specimen labels. Compliance will likely affect laboratory accreditation in future years by The Joint Commission and College of American Pathologists.

1-D Symbology

Still regarded as the standard by many, 1-D symbologies eventually may be replaced by 2-D. 1-D bar codes, however, are still used frequently in most laboratories. These symbologies require a larger space on labels, have higher error detection rates (even minor bar code defacement can cause scan errors), and have fewer data density capabilities. The most prevalent and standard 1-D symbology used in laboratories is Code 128; due to its 3 subtypes (A, B, and C) that can encode all 128 characters of American Standard Code for Information Interchange (ASCII) (all alphanumeric characters, upper and lowercase, 0–99). Each Code 128 bar code can shift between its 3 subtypes, which allows for a high character density to be encoded and reduces errors with a checksum. Code 128 is used by the International Society of Blood Transfusion (ISBT) for the ISBT 128 standard and has largely replaced the older blood bank Codabar bar code. Codabar was one of the first symbologies to incorporate error detection schema, thereby reducing the need for a discrete check digit.[12]

2-D Symbology

In the 1990s, with the mass production of charge-coupled devices (CCDs), scanner manufacturers were able to depend on 2-D scanning. These scanners use complex image analysis algorithms to decode 2-D symbologies, with better detection rates. In recent years, 2-D bar codes have seen increasing use in laboratories. They are scalable, require less label space, can encode much higher character densities, and have significantly decreased error detection rates; a 30% defacement of a 2-D bar code surface area can still be read. The 2-D symbology that has shown the most rapid adoption in laboratories is DataMatrix (**Fig. 2**). Depending on the matrix size and coding schema, DataMatrix can code up to 3116 numeric characters, 2335 alphanumeric characters, or 1555 bytes of binary data. This delivers more efficient encoding of ASCII characters into a fixed set of data. The ASCII string and error correction system are encoded into the bar code based on a specific algorithm that places all data into particular positions of the matrix. The initial installments of DataMatrix codes used convolutional error correction (referenced as ECC-000 to ECC-140). A more recent second subset of DataMatrix codes (recommended standard ECC-200), however, uses Reed-Solomon (RS) error correction techniques (allowing for correct reading even when a portion of the bar code is defaced), which has error detection rates in the Six Sigma confidence interval range. To further lower error detection rates, check digits have been incorporated in the encoded character sequence used concurrently with DataMatrix's RS error correction, diminishing error rates to as low as 1 in 10^{15} scan events.[12,15,16]

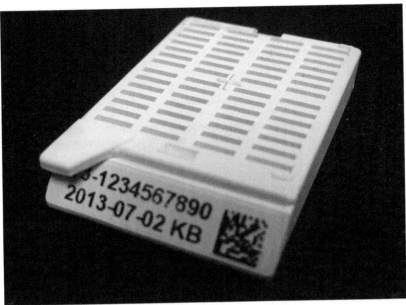

Fig. 2. Sample 2-D DataMatrix symbology printed on a white cassette. Bar code placement on the opposite side of the upper cassette lip enables easier access for scanners.

Another 2-D symbology, quick response (QR) code, has seen widespread adoption in all areas of the world. QR codes can encode up to 7089 numeric characters or 4296 alphanumeric characters. Similar to DataMatrix codes, they have high data density capabilities and RS error reduction techniques. QR codes have different versions, related to physical size, and 4 error correction levels (L, M, Q, and H). The variables that regulate the amount of data stored in a QR code include data type, version (smallest, 1; largest, 40), and error correction level. PDF417 is another 2-D symbology that is used in hazardous material labeling, storing technical specifications and calibration data on electronic instruments, and encoding civilian data on drivers' licenses. These codes can store up to approximately 1800 printable ASCII characters or 1100 binary characters. These are unique such that large data sets can be split into multiple organized PDF417 codes.[10,15]

ERROR RATES

A major advantage of implementing a bar coding and tracking system is the opportunity to eliminate labeling errors and achieve optimal patient safety, consequently reducing adverse events. Pathology studies have shown that up to 1% of manually labeled specimens and up to 72% of adverse events have problems related to specimen identification.[17–20] Other pathology studies identified that the greatest percentage of misidentification occurred at grossing.[21–23] Implementing bar-coding and tracking solutions in anatomic pathology laboratories can help minimize such errors **(Fig. 3)**.[24,25] Bar code error tolerance rates are high, which makes their use many fold more dependable than manual logging. Bar codes are robust tools that have created vast efficiency in identification and traceability of assets. With proper implementation of a bar code and tracking system, virtually all errors can be avoided. Data from the Henry Ford Hospital reported a 62% decrease of overall

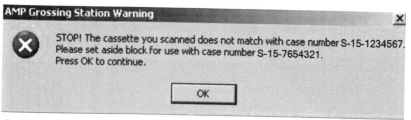

Fig. 3. Warning for improperly scanned cassette. The cassette for case S-15-7654321 was scanned while the specimen S-15-1234567 was previously scanned and opened.

misidentification case rate, 92% decrease in slide misidentification defects, and 125% increased technical throughput at their microtomy workstations after bar codes were introduced.[26]

BAR CODE FAILURES

Bar codes are not without fault (see **Fig. 2**).[27] Using pattern recognition, bar code scanners can identify code. Position finders can be found at the start/stop patterns of the opening and closing bars in a 1-D code or 3 bull's-eye corners of a QR code (or outer L shape of DataMatrix). The most common reason for bar code read failures is quiet zone violations. The quiet zone is the blank margin directly at the sides or around the periphery of the bar code; it is used to isolate the code of interest and ensure transfer of information of only the code being scanned. Bar code standards require a quiet zone of 10 times the smallest bar width, or 0.1 inch, whichever is largest. It has been shown, however, that most bar code readers do not work well if the quiet zone is less than 0.25 inches.[10,15]

Although bar codes are robust, there are a few reasons for why a bar code may fail (**Table 2**). Bar codes should be read accurately, quickly, and consistently.

- An intermittent read failure may result when a bar code scanner does not readily detect a code and continues to use signal processing algorithms to have a delayed correct read or, alternatively, may have a misread. Reasons for potential intermittent read failures are maximum print head dot density, typically measured in lines per inch or dots per inch, maximum printed media reproduction fidelity, and maximum spatial density of a scanning image.
- A misread failure occurs when a bar code is inappropriately read, where a new en-coded string represents a valid bar code sequence but not the intended sequence of the scanned bar code. These errors can be produced via bar code defacement or other defects while printing, from inadequate error detection methods, or from optical-mechanical scanner defects. Misread failures, if not prevented, may lead to serious adverse effects due to the difficulty in detecting this error.

Table 2
Types of bar code reader failures

Bar Code Failures	Description	Potential Harm
Intermittent read failure	Delayed scanner read	May lead to misread or delayed correct read
Nonread failure	Bar code not read	Least harm because bar code is not read
Misread failure	Inaccurate read	Most harm if not detected

- Nonread failures occur when a bar code is effectively defaced to the point of nonrecognition by a scanner and can no longer be decoded. These failures are readily identified because no data are decoded from an illegible bar code.

Bar code defacement is likely to occur in a histology laboratory, where bar codes are exposed to blades, heat, harsh chemicals, and microwaves. As discussed previously, this may lead to nonread or misread failures. To thwart these failures, bar codes have an intrinsic design to allow for redundancy. These redundancy factors exist in both 1-D and 2-D symbologies. The greater the height of a 1-D bar code, the greater is its redundancy factor. For instance, if a 1-D bar code has a hole punched in it, scanning at a different level where the code is complete likely still ensures accurate scanning. 2-D symbologies have more sophisticated redundancy factors, where the data are placed in several areas of the code, such that localized defacement unlikely prevents an accurate scan of the bar code.[10]

Another error correction technology that bar codes implement is a checksum. This uses an algorithm to calculate all numeric values of each character in the bar code string to a final summation value. The check digit is usually the last number on the 1-D symbologies and it must correlate with the checksum. Bar code scanning hardware and software must utilize this feature to corroborate that the checksum and check digit are correct to ensure successful decoding of the code; and safeguard against a potential misread. Checksums are largely represented, however, on 1-D and older symbologies. Newer and more robust error detection strategies, such as redundancy checking, have since been developed.

MEDIA AND LABELS

Other factors that may affect bar code readability stem from incompatible scanners, printing defects, or the media used to print the bar code/label itself. For instance, when a printer head malfunctions, due to wear and tear, it may not properly transfer heat to the printing media. Lengthy archival times may also have an impact on the durability of labels. Clinical Laboratory Improvement Amendments mandates that laboratories retain paraffin blocks for a minimum of 2 years, cytology slides for a minimum of 5 years, and histopathology slides for a minimum of 10 years.[28] It is, therefore, suggested that the selected media be tested to sustain at least 10 times the allotted storage time to account for thermal changes or other media transfer failures. It is important to select reliable media marker technologies that ideally endure many years. Because bar codes must remain on their assets somewhat indefinitely, their indelibility or impossibility of being removed or washed away is of prime importance. During the life cycle of histology slides and blocks, they experience significant time with abrasive chemical solvents and high temperatures. High temperatures may darken direct thermal labels or cause label adhesive to detach. Darkened labels may render bar code symbology illegible.[10] Hence, before investing in labels it is recommended to run several trials of printed labels through a rigorous histology workflow (eg, 72-hour xylene test or 1 week in a 65°C slide dryer) to demonstrate label fidelity.

STANDARDIZATION

Due to advancements in technology and the variety of bar code formats and systems available, complete standardization remains a challenge. For example, legacy bar code symbologies may still be used in older blood banks that need to deal with both Codabar and ISBT 128. A not-for-profit organization, GS1, has provided comprehensive standards for bar code numbers on a global scale. European, Asian, and

Australian countries now use a European Article Number bar code (13 digits) whereas the United States and Canada use UPC bar codes (12 digits). CLSI has developed laboratory standards for bar codes and labeling, which are available in their publications, AUTO02-A2, AUTO04-A (Laboratory Automation: Systems Operational Requirements, Characteristics, and Information Elements), and AUTO12-A (**Fig. 4**).[13,14,29] Hitherto, there were no set regulations to direct laboratory personnel when designing specimen labels, bar coding assets, or tracking specimens. AUTO12-A explains the required human-readable elements, locations, fonts, and font sizes needed on specimen labels. This standard also offers details about label size and layout and identifies Code 128 as the symbology to be used.[14] Continued focus on standardizing bar coding and specimen labels in anatomic pathology is still required. Lack of interoperability hinders sharing of assets between institutions and possibly locks laboratories in, preventing them from using existing bar codes on newer devices, such as automated immunostainers or whole-slide imaging scanners.

Bar coding reduces slide mislabeling.[30] Interinstitutional consultations remain problematic because laboratories are usually unable to read foreign bar codes (eg, bar codes generated by another laboratory). Solutions to address this problem, however, are starting to emerge. Certain LISs support foreign bar codes. This capability is available mainly for clinical laboratories. Hence, when an outside client sends samples with bar-coded identifiers already affixed, if the foreign bar code can be read, this prevents the need to relabel the specimen. In anatomic pathology, the traditional practice of handling consult materials (slides, blocks, specimen containers, and accompanying paperwork) involves manually staff relabeling these assets on arrival, which may lead to clerical errors. One solution is to apply temporary slide and/or cassette labels that are easily removed without defacing the consulting laboratory's underlying label (**Fig. 5**). These labels can be easily removed when materials are returned to the primary facility.

HARDWARE

As technology advanced, newer models of bar-code readers, printers, and computers became available. With the advent of CCD sensors, bar-code readers were able to utilize 2-D bar coding on a large, economical scale. 2-D bar codes are smaller, encode higher data density, and include better error correction methodologies, which make

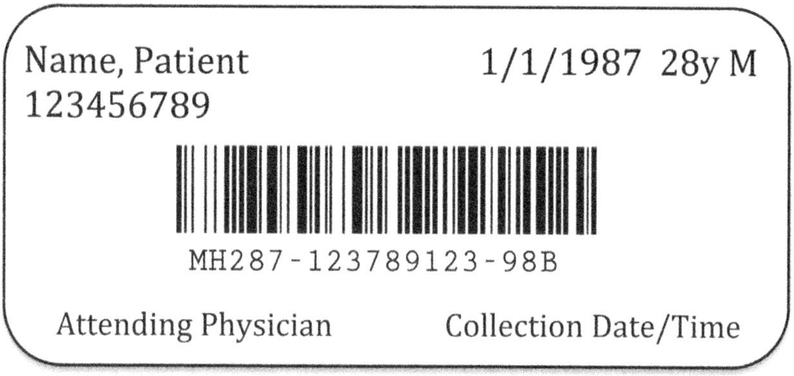

Fig. 4. AUTO12-A compliant label layout. Instead of the bar code as the most superior data element, the patient name is situated in the upper left corner in landscape format.

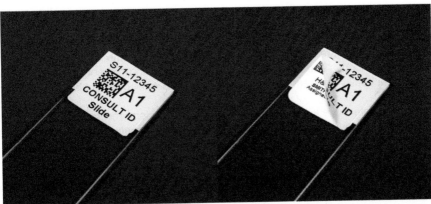

Fig. 5. Piggyback labeling of a glass slide for a consultation case. New labels that are easily removable are placed over existing labels and avoid the need to stick them on the opposite glass surface. (*Courtesy of* General Data Healthcare; with permission).

them ideal for labels that require less space on assets. Each bar code reader in an anatomic pathology laboratory is typically connected to an individual computer. Depending on the workflow, therefore, wherever bar codes need to be scanned, a computer system needs to be in place (eg, accessioning, grossing stations, tissue processors, microtomy, staining, slide assembly, slide distribution, and pathologist workstations). Adequate computers and network bandwidth to sustain these laboratory operations are necessary for smooth workflow.

Bar code readers by default are enabled to detect a wide array of symbologies; hence, configuration of these readers may be needed to recognize certain bar codes or to negate symbologies not used in the laboratory. Different bar code readers are available, including contact wands, laser bar code scanners, and image-based (camera) bar code readers. Scanners can be wired, wireless, or fixed/mounted. Omnidirectional scanners are preferred to single-line laser scanners because they can read symbologies in any orientation.[10]

Bar code printers are essential for labeling specimen containers, cassettes, and slides. Labels usually need to include bar codes as well as other patient identification information (case accession number, patient name, slide number, and so forth). Printing can be performed on an adhesive label or directly onto the cassette or slide. Bar code printing technology includes impact (dot matrix) and nonimpact (ink-jet, laser, and thermal) printing (**Table 3**).[15]

- Dot matrix printers print bar codes as a construct of numerous dots. These printers are the least expensive but have the lowest scanner readability.

Table 3
Comparison of bar code printer technology

Printer	Cost	Print Quality	Scanner Readability
Dot matrix	$	Good	Good
Ink-jet	$$$	Better	Good
Laser	$$	Better	Better
Thermal	$$	Best	Best

- Ink-jet printers have high output capabilities but suffer from inconsistent print quality and readability on different materials. Certain materials may cause the media to diffuse and render a bar code illegible.
- Laser printers create electrostatic energy to attract ions in the ink to the necessary areas of bar codes and are bonded together by heat and pressure. These printers have high quality and readability but often cannot be used with chemical resistant labels.
- Thermal printers use a series of chemical reactions to form rows of dots as the media passes through the heating printhead. Thermal transfer has improved using specialized inked ribbon. These bar code printers have excellent long-lasting print quality and scanner readability but are more costly than other printers.

SOFTWARE

Software is an integral piece of bar coding and tracking systems. Solutions currently exist as either a component the LIS, third-party vendor middleware, or custom-built tracking solutions.[31] The key to success is to properly interface the software with the LIS and all laboratory instruments to be used. Software systems may have most, but not all, desired asset tracking attributes. Laboratories may use software as is, contract with their vendor for additional support, obtain third-party software, or custom develop sought-after tools in-house. This may be hampered by proprietary systems that do not integrate seamlessly with existing LISs or other tracking solutions. Some laboratories have implemented a dual bar code system for this purpose. The ideal tracking software should be user friendly, be easily configurable with diverse options, and have the ability to be used on multiple computer platforms (eg, desktop, tablet, and touch-screen devices). Testing software compatibility should be trialed extensively to identify workflow amity.

WORKFLOW

Workflow should be analyzed to create a streamlined set of operations that produce the highest yield in the fewest steps. When implementing a new tracking system, it may be necessary to adjust workflow as needed. Specimen tracking should ideally start when a specimen is obtained from a patient (eg, in a doctor's office or operating room). This requires, however, bedside, operating room, and/or outreach remote printers and in-depth integration of the electronic medical record (in which orders accompanying the specimen are placed) and the LIS. Such labels could be placed on specimen containers and be preaccessioned in an LIS long before reaching a pathology laboratory. Tracking of patient assets for most anatomic pathology laboratories usually begins at the accessioning stage, using manual logs as the traceable record of custody during specimen procurement. At the time of accessioning, labels are printed when the case gets activated. It is at this time that some laboratories may also choose to print a predetermined number of cassettes, depending on the specimen type. Accessioners should be made aware of preprinting, sorting, and distribution errors. Otherwise, just-in-time printing should be deferred until the time of grossing.[12]

All patient specimen labels must be accurate and coincide with each asset (eg, container, cassette, or slide) for that patient. Bar coding can be used to audit and track each step in an anatomic pathology laboratory (**Fig. 6**), creating soft stops that require an asset bar code to be scanned before proceeding with each successive step (eg, microtomy, staining, slide distribution, sign-out, and transcription). When scanning a bar code at microtomy, the system should be able to automatically identify the case

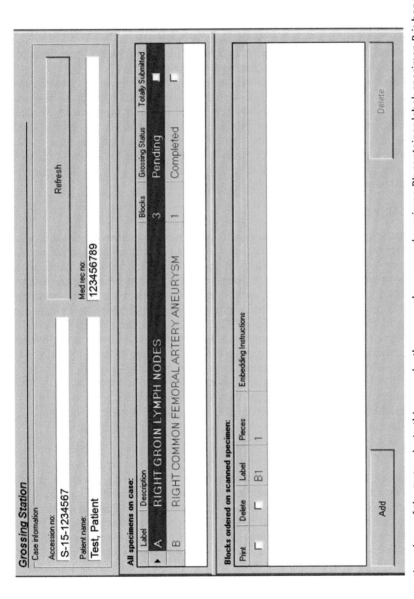

Fig. 6. Grossing station phase of the test cycle. In this example, the grosser has scanned specimen B's container label; specimen B is hence highlighted green. One cassette has been ordered and scanned (B1). Specimen A has not yet been scanned; however, 3 cassettes have been preordered.

and display ordered instructions (cut on edge, cross section, and so forth) and any other special orders to help drive workflow (use charged slides, send slides to immunohistochemistry, and so forth). This requires training laboratory personnel to use the system and how/when to scan bar codes. Although this may create additional steps when scanning these assets, overall it saves back-end time and energy when tracking a particular asset, if needed. Each scanned entry can record the time and workstation location where the asset was scanned and who was logged into the LIS at the time for this case, which is documented in the software for easy retrieval. Ongoing success depends on laboratory staff compliance and the capability of the tracking system to permit exceptions to be handled to avoid workarounds.

Workflow can be facilitated by using color-coding of stat specimens and/or specimens assigned to various subspecialties. There are numerous color cassettes available. For example, some laboratories choose to use red cassettes to indicate priority processing or designate tan to identify resident grossed specimens. Color-coding labels offers another option. It is recommended that all bar-code readers and labels be tested beforehand for machine-readable legibility to identify bar code readers that may have difficulty reading bar codes on select colors. Bar codes are often hard to read on dark red- or aqua-colored cassettes.

DASHBOARDS/STATUS MONITORS

Dashboards, or status monitors, are visual, tabular representations of scanned assets in the tracking system. They can be used to analyze workflow to identify areas of improvement or to check on the status of assets. For instance, with a quick glance at a dashboard, users can check to easily determine what time a specimen was accessioned, grossed, processed, embedded, cut, or stained or if the completed slides of a given case are assembled and ready for distribution. Users can audit case distribution and workload volume (**Fig. 7**). Each tracked step can display the length of time needed dealing with an asset. Each workstation with a bar code reader can be used as a soft stop. The more stops involved, the more granular the data on the dashboard (**Fig. 8**). Priority assignments can be segregated by flags or colors, or colors can be used to display delayed cases. Distribution of information on a dashboard can be sent out as quality measures via spreadsheets in an e-mail on the Web or publicly displayed on large monitors in a histology laboratory. These monitors can display up-to-date information, which promotes real-time tracking.[12,32]

IMPLEMENTATION

Until recently, many anatomic pathology laboratories traditionally used manual logging systems to track their cases. In such laboratories, implementing a tracking system usually involves radical changes. Planning should begin long before any particular solution is pursued. The exact how, where, and when specimen assets are tracked and what the data will be used for must be carefully planned. More specifically, it is important to perform an analysis of existing versus desired workflow, select labels, determine space availability for devices, and develop a downtime strategy as well as garner what degree of IT support and finances is needed.[12] After the preliminary assessment is made, choosing a vendor tracking solution is the next step, keeping in mind the goal of maintaining interoperability with what already exists in a laboratory (eg, LIS, instruments, and computers). Although several solutions have been developed, each laboratory likely needs individual configuration of its tracking solution. Field-testing of instruments, labels, various bar-code symbologies, and hardware is useful to demonstrate suitability and forecast potential integration

Event Time	Accession No	Material Description	Event Description	Event Location
07/23/2014 10:12:22 AM	S-14-321	Specimen A MEDIAL MARGIN OF THE RIGHT LEG MASS	Scanned by HANNA, MATTHEW.	Peds-grossing
07/23/2014 10:12:40 AM	S-14-321	Block A1 PROCESS AND EMBED A PARAFFIN BLOCK	Block verified by HANNA, MATTHEW.	Peds-grossing
07/23/2014 10:13:00 AM	S-14-321	Specimen B DISTAL MARGIN OF THE RIGHT LEG MASS	Scanned by HANNA, MATTHEW.	Peds-grossing
07/23/2014 10:13:18 AM	S-14-321	Block B1 PROCESS AND EMBED A PARAFFIN BLOCK	Block verified by HANNA, MATTHEW.	Peds-grossing
07/23/2014 10:13:37 AM	S-14-321	Specimen C DEEP MARGIN OF THE RIGHT LEG MASS	Scanned by HANNA, MATTHEW.	Peds-grossing
07/23/2014 10:13:57 AM	S-14-321	Block C1 PROCESS AND EMBED A PARAFFIN BLOCK	Block verified by HANNA, MATTHEW.	Peds-grossing
07/23/2014 10:14:20 AM	S-14-321	Specimen D PROXIMAL MARGIN OF THE RIGHT LEG MASS	Scanned by HANNA, MATTHEW.	Peds-grossing
07/23/2014 10:14:43 AM	S-14-321	Block D1 PROCESS AND EMBED A PARAFFIN BLOCK	Block verified by HANNA, MATTHEW.	Peds-grossing
07/23/2014 10:15:04 AM	S-14-321	Specimen E LATERAL MARGIN OF THE RIGHT LEG MASS	Scanned by HANNA, MATTHEW.	Peds-grossing
07/23/2014 10:15:23 AM	S-14-321	Block E1 PROCESS AND EMBED A PARAFFIN BLOCK	Block verified by HANNA, MATTHEW.	Peds-grossing
07/23/2014 10:15:46 AM	S-14-321	Specimen F SUPERFICIAL MARGIN OF THE RIGHT LEG M....	Scanned by HANNA, MATTHEW.	Peds-grossing
07/23/2014 10:16:04 AM	S-14-321	Block F1 PROCESS AND EMBED A PARAFFIN BLOCK	Block verified by HANNA, MATTHEW.	Peds-grossing
07/25/2014 3:47:30 PM	A-14-123	Specimen B PLACENTA	Scanned by HANNA, MATTHEW.	Grossing-GI Station
07/25/2014 3:47:40 PM	A-14-123	Block B1 Resident Block	Block verified by HANNA, MATTHEW.	Grossing-GI Station
07/25/2014 3:47:44 PM	A-14-123	Block B2 Resident Block	Block verified by HANNA, MATTHEW.	Grossing-GI Station
07/25/2014 3:47:49 PM	A-14-123	Block B3 Resident Block	Block verified by HANNA, MATTHEW.	Grossing-GI Station
07/25/2014 3:47:53 PM	A-14-123	Block B4 Resident Block	Block verified by HANNA, MATTHEW.	Grossing-GI Station
07/25/2014 3:47:58 PM	A-14-123	Block B5 Resident Block	Block verified by HANNA, MATTHEW.	Grossing-GI Station
07/25/2014 3:48:03 PM	A-14-123	Block B6 Resident Block	Block verified by HANNA, MATTHEW.	Grossing-GI Station
07/25/2014 3:48:07 PM	A-14-123	Block B7 Resident Block	Block verified by HANNA, MATTHEW.	Grossing-GI Station
01/19/2015 8:40:15 PM	S-15-282	Specimen C LEFT PELVIC LYMPH NODE	Scanned by HANNA, MATTHEW.	Grossing-GYN

Fig. 7. Workstation user audit. This inquiry allows all scan events by a user to be identified in real time, displaying the event time, case (accession) number, specimen, user, and location.

	Processing History					
Performed On	Action Name	Material ID	Action D&T	Employee	Site	Workst
Specimen	Specimen Collected		3/5/2015 11:23 AM	HANNA, MATTHEW	m	HACC1
Specimen	Specimen Collected		3/5/2015 11:23 AM	HANNA, MATTHEW	m	HACC1
Material	Material Received	MS-15-204-A	3/5/2015 11:23 AM	HANNA, MATTHEW	m	HACC1
Specimen	Specimen Received		3/5/2015 11:23 AM	HANNA, MATTHEW	m	HACC1
Order	Order Inserted		3/5/2015 11:23 AM	HANNA, MATTHEW	m	HACC1
Material	PRINT CASSETTES	MS-15-204-A	3/5/2015 11:27 AM	HANNA, MATTHEW	m	HACC1
Specimen	Gross Description Modified		3/5/2015 11:29 AM	HANNA, MATTHEW	m	GROS1
Material	Grossing	MS-15-204-A	3/5/2015 11:29 AM	HANNA, MATTHEW	m	GROS1
Material	Grossing Complete- Scan block	MS-15-204-A1	3/5/2015 11:29 AM	HANNA, MATTHEW	m	GROS1
Material	RBS - Store Material in Storage	MS-15-204-A	3/5/2015 11:29 AM	HANNA, MATTHEW	m	HACC1
Material	ASSIGN AND LOAD CASSETTES IN TISSUE PROC	MS-15-204-A1	3/5/2015 11:29 AM	HANNA, MATTHEW	m	TISPR1
Material	SEND SPECIMEN TO STORAGE	MS-15-204-A	3/5/2015 11:29 AM	HANNA, MATTHEW	m	HACC1
Material	Specimen Storage Check In	MS-15-204-A	3/5/2015 11:29 AM	HANNA, MATTHEW	m	HACC1
Material	ASSIGN TISSUE PROCESSOR	MS-15-204-A1	3/5/2015 11:29 AM	HANNA, MATTHEW	m	TISPR1
Material	BLOCK EMBEDDING	MS-15-204-A1	3/5/2015 11:29 AM	HANNA, MATTHEW	m	EMBD1
Material	Microtomy	MS-15-204-A1	3/5/2015 11:40 AM	HANNA, MATTHEW	m	MCR1
Panel Slide S1	Microtomy	MS-15-204-A1	3/5/2015 11:40 AM	HANNA, MATTHEW	m	MCR1
Material	BLOCKS TO FILE	MS-15-204-A1	3/5/2015 11:40 AM	HANNA, MATTHEW	m	HACC1
Panel Slide S1	Slide Stain	MS-15-204-A1	3/5/2015 11:41 AM	HANNA, MATTHEW	m	STA1
Panel Slide S1	CASE DISTRIBUTION	MS-15-204-A1	3/5/2015 11:41 AM	HANNA, MATTHEW	m	DIST1
Final Interpret...	Order Interpreted		3/5/2015 4:17 PM	HERZFELD, EMILY	m	PATH2
Interpretation	N - RBS - Assign interpretation for Preview		3/5/2015 4:27 PM	HERZFELD, EMILY	m	PATH2
Final Interpret...	Final Report Signed Out		3/5/2015 4:31 PM	HERZFELD, EMILY	m	PATH2

Fig. 8. Case processing history. Audit trail of different workstations, tracking a single case through the laboratory workflow (specimen collection to final case interpretation).

difficulties. Frequent discussions with vendors or hired consultants hopefully address any issues that arise. Implementation from the time of deployment to training requires support from informatics and IT staff, personnel (end users) in the laboratory, pathologists, and senior administration.[33]

INVENTORY MANAGEMENT SYSTEMS

Inventory of a pathology laboratory may include a plethora of items. To control the supply and demand of such supplies, inventory management systems have been developed, either as a stand-alone product or as part of an LIS. The focus of these systems is to assimilate product identification, asset tracking, and order management. Manually logging items in a pathology laboratory is a tremendous burden and importantly more prone to errors. These systems help ensure appropriate availability of reagents, cassettes, glass slides, personal protective equipment, and so forth. Important directives to establish include product lists, monthly usage, frequency of ordering, storage, expiration dates, and cost. Systems have been developed to alert or automatically order new supplies when inventory runs low. Having a constant supply of supplies in a pathology laboratory is vital for an efficient operation. Shared resource facilities (eg, tissue biorepository) may greatly benefit from such inventory management systems.[34]

FUTURE DIRECTIONS

RFID is an emerging but recently introduced technology in pathology (**Table 4**).[35,36] RFID is a method of uniquely identifying items using radio wave signals emitted from an RFID tag that are detected by a reader with an antenna. These tags can encode data about an asset but do not always necessitate user action to physically scan the tag. Where bar codes fall short of only allowing individual static data to be encoded, RFID tags have the ability to allow multiple dynamic data updates, with rapid read rates and batch readability. Radio frequencies can penetrate nonmetallic objects. In laboratories, RFID tags can be placed on each specimen/asset to be traced. RFID tags exist in passive or active forms, where passive tags draw electromagnetic energy from the radio waves of a reader, and active tags have their own power source. Active tags are battery powered, enabling longer read ranges (up to 100 m); however, this limits their longevity for assets being archived or for use in tissue repository laboratories. Passive tags have shorter read ranges (less than 25 m) and a reported life

Table 4
Comparison of bar code and radiofrequency identification technologies

	Bar Code		Radiofrequency Identification		
	1-D	2-D	Passive	Active	Near-field Communication
Data density	Low	Intermediate	High	High	High
Line of site	Required	Required	None	None	None
Manual or automated	Manual	Manual	Automated	Automated	Automated
Batch capability	No	No	Yes	Yes	Yes
Frequency interferences	None	None	More sensitive	Less sensitive	Less sensitive
Battery requirement	None	None	None	Yes	None
Read vs read-write	Read	Read	Read-write	Read-write	Read-write

span of approximately 20 years. Active tags are also larger and cost more. Tags can be preserialized, programmable, or both. Preserialized tags are preprogrammed at the time of manufacturing and are assigned a unique sequential character sequence. Programmable tags are encoded at the time of use by the user. RFID technology is currently more expensive than bar codes. Also, few vendors offer them as a part of their tracking solution.[10,37] RFID tags have been shown to be resilient in anatomic pathology laboratories.[38] It is likely that RFID technology will be increasingly used in laboratories in the near future.

NFC has been recently popularized in smartphone technology related to contactless payment systems. NFC is a specialized subset of RFID technology. RFID frequencies exist as low (<0.3 MHz), high (3–30 MHz), ultrahigh (860–950 MHz), and microwave (2450–5800 MHz) ranges.[37] NFC technology operates at the same high frequency range (predominantly 13.56 MHz) as other RFID tags; however, its distinguishing factor is that an NFC-labeled item can serve as a reader and a tag simultaneously. Depending on the frequency, RFID tags can be read at far or near distances, NFC technology is built to have secure reads at only a few centimeters. It is anticipated that similar technology will likely be used to improve tracking in health care, including pathology.[39–42]

SUMMARY

Anatomic pathology laboratories have a responsibility to modernize and sustain increasing efficiency, leverage automation, and foster patient safety. Misidentification errors in laboratories have the capability to cause devastating events. The use of bar coding and tracking systems for anatomic pathology laboratories has, therefore, become common. Although workflow changes may incorporate dramatic reforms, this technology has the ability to decrease laboratory blunders while proportionately increasing efficiency. As technology has advanced, more robust products and innovative solutions have been witnessed. As with the introduction of 2-D high data density bar codes in laboratories, RFID technology offers similar promising benefits.

REFERENCES

1. Becich MJ, Gilbertson JR, Gupta D, et al. Pathology and patient safety: the critical role of pathology informatics in error reduction and quality initiatives. Clin Lab Med 2004;24(4):913–43.
2. Sharma G, Parwani AV, Raval JS, et al. Contemporary issues in transfusion medicine informatics. J Pathol Inform 2011;2:3.
3. Richmond L. Barcoding in the lab: achieving error-free efficiencies. Healthc Inform 1994;11:26–30.
4. Snyder SR, Favoretto AM, Derzon JH, et al. Effectiveness of barcoding for reducing patient specimen and laboratory testing identification errors: a Laboratory Medicine Best Practices systematic review and meta-analysis. Clin Biochem 2012;45(13–14):988–98.
5. Pagliaro P, Turdo R, Capuzzo E. Patients' positive identification systems. Blood Transfus 2009;7:313–8.
6. Morrison AP, Tanasijevic MJ, Goonan EM, et al. Reduction in specimen labeling errors after implementation of a positive patient identification system in phlebotomy. Am J Clin Pathol 2010;133:870–7.
7. ID History. Progression of proposed product ID symbols. ID History Museum. 2013. Available at: http://www.idhistory.com/. Accessed January 17, 2015.

8. Ashford P, Distler P, Gee A, et al. ISBT 128 implementation plan for cellular therapy products. J Clin Apher 2007;22(5):258–64.
9. Butch S, Distler P, Georgsen J, et al. ISBT 128: an introduction. 3rd edition. 2006. Available at: http://www.transfusionmedicine.ca/sites/transfusionmedicine/files/articles/ISBT%20128_Attachments/ISBT%20an%20Introduction.pdf. Accessed January 18, 2015.
10. Balis UJ, Pantanowitz L. Specimen tracking and identification systems. In: Pantanowitz L, Balis UJ, Tuthill JM, editors. Pathology informatics: theory & practice. Chicago: ASCP Press; 2012. p. 283–304.
11. Specification for bar code symbols, vol. MH10.8M-1983. ANSI; 1983.
12. Pantanowitz L, Mackinnon AC Jr, Sinard JH. Tracking in anatomic pathology. Arch Pathol Lab Med 2013;137:1798–810.
13. Mountain PJ, Callaghan JV, Chou D, et al. Laboratory automation: bar codes for specimen container identification; approved standard. In: CLSI document AUTO02-A2, vol. 25, 2nd edition. Wayne (PA): CLSI; 2005. p. 25.
14. Hawker CD, Agrawal Y, Balis UJ, et al. Specimen labels: content and location, fonts, and label orientation; approved standard. In: CLSI document AUTO12-A, vol. 31, 1st edition. Wayne (PA): CLSI; 2011. p. 48.
15. Palmer RC. The bar code book: a comprehensive guide to reading, printing, specifying, evaluating, and using bar code and other machine readable symbols. 5th edition. Victoria, BC, Canada: Trafford Publishing; 2007.
16. Cowan DF. Bar coding in the laboratory. In: Cowan DF, editor. Informatics for the clinical laboratory: a practical guide for the pathologist. New York: Springer; 2005. p. 156–68.
17. Lippi G, Blanckaert N, Bonini P, et al. Causes, consequences, detection, and prevention of identification errors in laboratory diagnostics. Clin Chem Lab Med 2009;47:143–53.
18. Nakhleh RE, Zarbo RJ. Surgical pathology specimen identification and accessioning: a College of American Pathologists Q-Probes Study of 1 004 115 cases from 417 institutions. Arch Pathol Lab Med 1996;120(3):227–33.
19. Dunn EJ, Moga PJ. Patient misidentification in laboratory medicine: a qualitative analysis of 227 root cause analysis reports in the Veterans Health Administration. Arch Pathol Lab Med 2010;134:244–55.
20. Valenstein PN, Sirota RL. Identification errors in pathology and laboratory medicine. Clin Lab Med 2004;24(4):979–96.
21. Nakhleh RE, Idowu MO, Souers RJ, et al. Mislabeling of cases, specimens, blocks, and slides: a College of American Pathologists study of 136 institutions. Arch Pathol Lab Med 2011;135(8):969–74.
22. Layfield LJ, Anderson GM. Specimen labeling errors in surgical pathology: an 18-month experience. Am J Clin Pathol 2010;134:466–70.
23. Nakhleh RE. Patient safety and error reduction in surgical pathology. Arch Pathol Lab Med 2008;132:181–5.
24. Simpson NJ, Kleinberg KA. Implementation guide to barcoding and auto-id in healthcare: improving quality and patient safety. Chicago: HIMSS; 2009.
25. Informatics for the Clinical Laboratory. A practical guide for the pathologist. New York: Springer; 2002. p. 156–68.
26. Zarbo RJ, Tuthill JM, D'Angelo R, et al. The henry ford production system: reduction of surgical pathology in-process misidentification defects by bar code- specified work process standardization. Am J Clin Pathol 2009;131(4):468–77.
27. Snyder ML, Carter A, Jenkins K, et al. Patient misidentifications caused by errors in standard barcode technology. Clin Chem 2010;56:1–7.

28. Eiseman E, Haga SB. Handbook of human tissue sources. Chapter 6 Pathology specimens, 1999. Available at: http://www.rand.org/content/dam/rand/pubs/monograph_reports/MR954/MR954.chap6.pdf. Accessed January 11, 2015.

29. Tomar RH, Aller RD, Arkin CF, et al. Laboratory automation: systems operational requirements, characteristics, and information elements; approved standard. In: CLSI document AUTO04-A, vol. 21, 1st edition. Wayne (PA): CLSI; 2001. p. 40.

30. Sharma G, Piccoli A, Kelly SM, et al. Reduction of anatomical pathology slide mislabel rate due to implementation of barcoding at two tertiary care hospitals. Mod Pathol 2011;24(Suppl 1):342A.

31. Sinard JH, Gershkovich P. Custom software development for use in a clinical laboratory. J Pathol Inform 2012;3:44.

32. Sinard JH, Mutnick N, Gershkovich P. Histology asset tracking dashboard: real-time monitoring and dynamic work lists. J Pathol Inform 2010;1:18.

33. Force HB. Implementation guide for the use of bar code technology in healthcare. Chicago: Healthcare Information and Management Systems Society; 2003.

34. Dash RC, Robb JA, Booker DL, et al. Biospecimens and biorepositories for the community pathologist. Arch Pathol Lab Med 2012;136(6):668–78.

35. Briggs L, Davis R, Gutierrez A, et al. RFID in the blood supply chain: increasing productivity, quality and patient safety. J Healthc Inf Manag 2009;23:54–63.

36. Knels R, Ashford P, Bidet F, et al. Guidelines for the use of RFID technology in transfusion medicine. Vox Sang 2010;98:1–24.

37. Lou JJ, Andrechak GA, Riben M, et al. A review of radio frequency identification technology for the anatomic pathology or biorepository laboratory: much promise, some progress, and more work needed. J Pathol Inform 2011;2:34.

38. Leung AA, Lou JJ, Mareninov S, et al. Tolerance testing of passive radio frequency identification tags for solvent, temperature, and pressure conditions encountered in an anatomic pathology or biorepository setting. J Pathol Inform 2010;1:21.

39. Swedberg C. Brigham and Women's Hospital Tests NFC RFID for patient bedsides. RFID Journal 2013. Available at: http://www.rfidjournal.com/articles/view?10511/. Accessed January 7, 2015.

40. Agrawal A. Medication errors: prevention using information technology systems. Br J Clin Pharmacol 2009;67:681–6.

41. Section of Pharmacy Informatics and Technology, American Society of Health-System Pharmacists. ASHP statement on bar-code-enabled medication administration technology. Am J Health Syst Pharm 2009;66:588–90.

42. Poon EG, Keohane CA, Yoon CS, et al. Effect of bar-code technology on the safety of medication administration. N Engl J Med 2010;362:1698–707.

Enhancing and Customizing Laboratory Information Systems to Improve/ Enhance Pathologist Workflow

Douglas J. Hartman, MD

KEYWORDS

- Image-embedded reports • Voice recognition • Pre–sign-out quality assurance
- Computerized provider order entry

OVERVIEW

The workflow for pathologists constitutes a broad category due to the many roles that surgical pathologists must engage in during a workday. These roles include interpreting histopathologic findings, generating a diagnostic report to clearly convey pathologic findings, communicating critical results when appropriate, ensuring quality of the pathology system, educating future pathologists (residents and fellows), and, when appropriate, having quality assurance performed on the diagnostic findings. To understand various ways that a pathologist's workflow can be enhanced, understanding the practice workflow for pathologists is critical.

Many academic practices and some community pathology practices have converted into a subspecialized sign-out service.[1–3] Several factors are contributing to this trend: (1) increased pressure for consolidation or concentration of hospital services into a centralized center, (2) increasing complexity of the knowledge base, and (3) requests from clinical colleagues for subspecialty expertise. There is variability among how the subspecialization works by practice, with most academic practices having pathologists dedicated to a single subspecialty whereas community practices may rely on subspecialty expertise in a consultative role for specific or difficult cases. A mixture of subspecialty-only pathologists with general pathologists is appealing from a management standpoint because caseload balancing can be readily performed when adjustable pathologist labor is possible, depending on the volume of a particular organ specimen type. With the ongoing health care changes, subspecialty expertise

This article originally appeared in Surgical Pathology Clinics, Volume 8, Issue 2, June 2015.
Disclosure Statement: author for one up-to-date on topic - Clinical Pathological Cases in Gastroenterology, otherwise no disclosures.
Department of Anatomic Pathology, University of Pittsburgh Medical Center, 200 Lothrop Street, A-607, Pittsburgh, PA 15213, USA
E-mail address: hartmandj@upmc.edu

Clin Lab Med 36 (2016) 31–39
http://dx.doi.org/10.1016/j.cll.2015.09.004
0272-2712/16/$ – see front matter © 2016 Elsevier Inc. All rights reserved.

labmed.theclinics.com

demand is likely to increase in order to deliver higher-quality, outcome-driven health care. Just as pathologists are becoming subspecialized, the clients that pathologists serve have been changing as well.

Clinical teams have become a mixture of attending physicians who themselves are becoming more and more subspecialized, house staff (fellows and residents), nurse practitioners or physician assistants, nurse coordinators, nurses, and so forth. The secondary team members are sometimes interacting with the pathology department more than the attending physician due to time constraints. Additionally, pathology reports have many different intended audiences—for instance, a surgical resection report is completed predominantly for the operating surgeon, but a primary care physician/oncologist/radiation oncologist (and so forth) may be interested in report content that differs from the surgeon. Additionally, greater transparency of records is demanded by the public, which is leading to surgical pathology reports going directly to the patients themselves. These challenges present an opportunity for pathology to demonstrate its contribution to the clinical team but the solutions often involve balancing various competing needs.

It is within this setting that pathologists must complete the many diverse tasks that are requested of them. Within this article, I discuss several possible ways to enhance/customize surgical pathology workflow. Many of these may be more helpful depending on the clinical practice setup.

VOICE RECOGNITION TECHNOLOGY

Several studies have explored the use of voice recognition technology in pathology with mixed interpretation of the results. One component to consider when looking at voice recognition is the current practice environment. If there is a delay between dictation and completion of reports, voice recognition technology is an attractive alternative. In a system where transcription completes reports quickly, however, the altered workflow associated with voice recognition is not welcomed because there is little gain compared with the prior system. Voice recognition technology is particularly suited to filling in template forms rather than generating a final (free text–based) diagnosis.[4] Henricks and colleagues[4] demonstrated that targeted deployment of voice recognition was cost effective (reduced 2 full-time equivalent positions and payback period was less than 2 years). Kang and colleagues[5] also found that voice recognition technology was amenable to use predominantly for gross description. The use of preprogrammed templates facilitated less text editing of the reports and allowed for greater acceptance.[5] Kang and colleagues[5] discussed several barriers to adoption of voice recognition technology for final diagnosis. These barriers boil down to a lack of standardization in pathology reporting.[5] The pathology department at State University of New York at Stony Brook adopted voice recognition for the complete surgical pathology workflow (from gross description to final diagnosis sign-out).[6] Although not explicitly stated in their study, this group seems to have experienced long turnaround time with their transcription service, and some pathologists submitted handwritten copies of reports to be transcribed.[6] Within this background, the investigators found voice recognition technology a marked improvement, but, despite its improvements over the prior system, some pathologists still used the prior system for report generation.[6]

WORK PROCESSING

Many articles have been written in recent years describing implementation of lean principles based on the Toyota Production System.[7] Other articles also describe efficient processing as the Henry Ford Production System.[8] These systems are largely taken from the manufacturing world. The systems describe changes to the workflow of a specimen of pathology into a continuous flow system. Although continuous flow systems reduce errors and are efficient, some steps in the processing of pathology specimens require batch processing. The biggest batch process for pathology specimen workflow is the specimen processors. Numerous articles have described implementation of continuous process flow to gross processing or continuous flow to slide generation but few if any studies have described a 100% continuous flow specimen processing system.[7–12] This may be because this physically cannot be done. Therefore, the processing of specimen has been turned into a mix of batch and continuous flow processes. Therefore, for a sign-out pathologist, considering an optimal workflow depends on the method for receiving the slide—continuous flow or batch processes. Theoretically, if a pathologist is receiving 1 slide every 10 minutes, then the pathologist can advance that case within a 10-minute window before the next slide comes out. Most departments, however, deliver slides in batches, leading to the pathologist working within a batch processing workflow. This process can include house staff also within the process, which can add another step in batch processing. In the future, with the introduction of whole-slide imaging into the workflow process, continuous flow may be more of a reality than can be achieved in practical terms now. A sample diagram of the workflow from slides leaving histology to report delivery to downstream end users within a pathology department is described in **Fig. 1**. Although continuous flow systems seem the most efficient method, batch processing is currently an integral component of the health care system.

To this end, new iterations of laboratory information systems (LIS) software have tested providing case status updates to sign-out pathologists, for instance, the cases accessioned, the cases of gross complete, and the cases of final diagnosis. Although it is difficult to know how this functionality will work from a practical standpoint, this functionality suggests that the dynamic process of specimen processing can be interactive. Some institutions have instituted specimen tracking through their LIS systems (see the article by Pantanowitz elsewhere in this issue).[13] This specimen tracking may also interact with the clinical systems from which specimens are received. The current workflow is less granular, but perhaps as bar coding expands, this functionality will become more granular. This type of system may also be helpful when whole-slide imaging is implemented (notification of scanning status for slides and so forth).

QUALITY ASSURANCE

Since the release of the Institute of Medicine 1999 report, "To Err is Human: Building a Safer Health System,"[14] several articles have been published describing quality assurance measures and proposing novel ways to insure quality in surgical pathology. Nakhleh[15] provided an excellent review of all aspects of quality in surgical pathology (see also the article by Nakhleh elsewhere in this issue). A simple representation of errors breaks them down into preanalytical, analytical, and postanalytical errors.[15] Pathologists can assist with identifying preanalytical and postanalytical errors but these errors are often influenced by conditions outside pathology's control. Pathologists are able to monitor and improve the analytical aspect of quality assurance for surgical pathology. Some proposed mechanisms to reduce errors include bar code processing of specimens by gross room staff and histology (see the article by Pantanowitz elsewhere in this issue). Several methods are used to perform peer review.[15] Many departments have installed second review of selected reports prior to sign-out whereas other departments have implemented random case selection prior to sign-out, facilitating rapid performance of quality assurance and real-time case feedback.[16] Regardless of the method

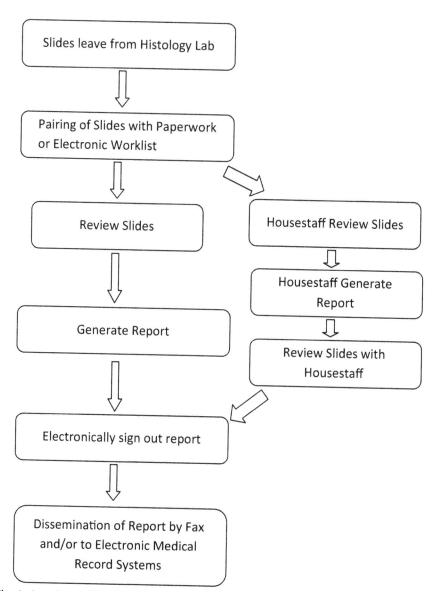

Fig. 1. Sample workflow for slides to report signout.

whereby a department determines quality assurance, the performance of quality assurance concurrent with the sign-out of a case provides benefits, including less time locating the case and potential to correct an error before it goes out in a report. A few studies have documented the benefit of pre–sign-out quality assurance.[16,17]

SURGICAL PATHOLOGY REPORT

The surgical pathology report is constantly under evolution as knowledge of diagnostic, therapeutic, and prognostic features is expanded. Increasing demands are placed to include more pathologic data in an era of personalized medicine.[18]

Histologic images embedded within surgical pathology reports have been possible for some time. This system of surgical pathology reporting has been provided predominantly by commercial pathology groups.[18] In my opinion, the lack of widespread adoption of whole-slide imaging systems and the difficulty of representing the pertinent pathologic findings in a single image have impeded more widespread adoption of image embedded surgical pathology reports. Additionally, the lack of transmission of images across interfaces within the electronic medical record and the lack of widespread color printing delivery of pathology reports (many reports are still delivered via fax) also impede the adoption of this method for reporting. Besides the increased use of images in reports, commercial laboratories also use templates with graphics and synoptics to enhance and market their pathology reports.[19,20]

Synoptic reporting, in particular for tumor staging, has been widely advocated. Synoptic reporting can be integrated with the LIS or via Web-based tools.[21–23] The benefits of synoptic reports include better report standardization and allow data to be stored as discrete data fields.[23] Storing synoptic data within discrete data fields within an LIS provides ready access to the data points for downstream systems (for instance, to tumor registries). The adoption of synoptic reporting can be used to replace the current narrative surgical report or as a supplement to it.[24] Ellis[24] suggests that "structured" reporting (such as synoptic reporting) may be an amenable solution to replace the current narrative surgical pathology reports. Ellis envisions structured reporting (such as synoptic reporting) to include a minimal dataset while allowing individual pathologists to supplement the description of the pathologic feature as appropriate.[24] In the United States, the Physician Quality Reporting System regulations have been implemented to encourage minimal data elements within surgical pathology reports—pathologic assessment of primary tumor stage (pT) and pathologic assessment of the involvement of regional lymph nodes (pN) stage for colorectal carcinoma, pT and pN stage for breast carcinoma, pT and pN stage for prostate carcinoma and the presence/absence of dysplasia when Barrett esophagus is identified; and quantitative HER2 evaluation by immunohistochemistry uses the system recommended by the American Society of Clinical Oncology/College of American Pathologists guidelines.[25] Without the creation of discrete data from either a synoptic or structured report, electronic health records will not be able to harness the potential for decision support and verification.

AUTOMATED ORDER ENTRY TO PATHOLOGY LABORATORY INFORMATION SYSTEMS

The introduction of computerized physician order entry (CPOE) has been driven largely to reduce medication-related errors.[26] The use of CPOE for laboratory test order entry provides an opportunity to improve laboratory test ordering efficiency, laboratory utilization, and patient care.[27] The benefits of CPOE in clinical pathology laboratory testing include reduced risk for mislabeled specimens, incorrect container types, lost requisitions, and incorrect testing.[27] CPOE is being introduced, however, into the surgical pathology system. This offers the ability to increase efficiency within the health care system; however, it leads to nonpathology workers entering information into the pathology LIS. Some of the benefits (such as incorrect testing and incorrect container types) associated with CPOE for clinical pathology laboratory testing do not apply to anatomic pathology. This change in the delivery of order to anatomic pathology will require pathology departments to educate the clinical administrative staff about the type of information needed to perform an appropriate pathologic examination. In the past, this task has been accomplished by requiring the completion of a requisition form, although the requirement of a requisition does not always mean all of the clinical information is provided.[28] One study of dermatopathology requisitions found no difference between hand-written requisitions (3.0%) and electronic requisitions (3.9%).[29] With the implementation of a CPOE system, the possibility of clinical decision support can be introduced[27]; however, it is unclear how clinical decision support systems would affect the performance of anatomic pathology services. Although clinical pathology laboratory is more advanced than the surgical pathology laboratory when it comes to electronic order entry, the current order entry systems do not support add-on testing (additional studies and so forth).[27]

USE OF IMAGES IN SURGICAL PATHOLOGY

It is said, "a picture can say a thousand words."[30] The possible uses of images within surgical pathology extend from scanning of documents (either outside reports or requisitions) to gross images to and microscopic images.

In recent years the advent of high throughput document scanning has created an opportunity to scan specimen requisitions into an LIS. One of the drawbacks of this ability is that it encourages hand-written orders that may be illegible (discussed previously regarding order entry as an alternative system). Even in an electronic order system, there may be a role for document scanning ability within the LIS, particularly for downtime procedures, additional/follow-up orders on specimens, or documentation of extradepartmental consultations. The image file type can be customized to contain specific properties related to the file extension—for instance, at the University of Pittsburgh Medical center, we have created a specific file type for requisitions, which allows for printing of the surgical pathology working draft along with the requisition. In this example, the need to match a requisition with the printed working draft (printed after the gross complete status was made) was eliminated because the file type from the case was matched when the case was ready to print the working draft. Some potential future directions might be to automate notification of the sign-out pathologist when additional tests have been requested or an extradepartmental consultation has been received. Within our department, as part of quality assurance, it is policy to issue an addendum statement when an outside consultation on a pathology report is received. Reduction of manual entry of documents via document scanning is ideal but unlikely to be completely eliminated in the current system.

Image documentation of gross abnormalities of surgical specimens may represent an alternative documentation of the type of specimen/gross findings received. It is our departmental policy to obtain gross images of surgical specimens. Given the expanded use of pathologist assistants for most grossing responsibilities, the images obtained sometimes may not be of optimal quality. One possible solution to encourage more optimal gross images is to integrate the image capture work into the gross description work. Currently, the acquisition of the image is one more task assigned to a pathologist assistant on top of other responsibilities. Integrating this into the workflow would encourage appropriate gross documentation and potentially reduce a pathologist assistant's time per case. If the gross measurements could be derived from the image, it might be possible to store these measurements as discrete values for later use within the LIS, for instance, in the generation of the final report or the completion of a synoptic report. This workflow is currently not possible and our pathologist assistants mostly generate narrative gross descriptions based on grossing manual or institutional guidelines on top of acquiring gross images of the surgical specimens.

The use of microscopic images within surgical pathology reports is discussed previously. With the lack of widespread whole-slide imaging devices, the acquisition of microscopic images is tedious. At the University of Pittsburgh Medical Center, using the same LIS software for microscopic image integration into the surgical pathology report, we have experimented with placing a 2-D bar code on surgical pathology reports. The 2-D bar code linked to a Web site with content related to the final diagnosis of the surgical pathology report (no diagnostic information was present within the link). The intent of this code would be to provide information to the end-user information above and beyond the diagnostic aspect of the surgical pathology report. At the University of Pittsburgh Medical Center, we have yet to assess the end-user viewpoint of this strategy but no feedback was directed after instituting this experiment. Several conclusions could be suggested by this small experiment: (1) paper reports are no longer the primary method by which end users access their surgical pathology reports, (2) end users focus only on the diagnostic part of the reports, or (3) there was no to limited novelty of having a 2-D bar code on the report. Within the past 10 years, there has been an expansion of electronic records from departments other than radiology or pathology. This change may reflect why a paper surgical pathology report no longer is used by end users. A recent article described a delayed identification of errors in dates associated with laboratory test reporting with the implementation of a new order entry system.[31] This likely reflects overworked clinical colleagues and a lack of awareness to pathology quality issues from clinical colleagues. One of the fundamentally most important functions for our surgical pathology reports is to communicate results to the end users.[32] To the extent that it is possible, this effort could represent a further method to communicate with clinical colleagues pertinent information to their practice or a given medical condition. Future directions for adding supplemental data will require coordination between the downstream clinical systems and the pathology LIS. This function might pair well with efforts to electronically order additional studies/tests on a surgical pathology specimen. Coded diagnostic information (such as the implementation of *International Classification of Diseases, Tenth Revision*) represents an increased granularity of medical coding and the potential to use this by pathology to supplement clinical decision support systems is vast.[33]

Pathologist workflow is affected by many different variables, predominantly related to the setup of the practice that they work for. Surgical pathologists are tasked with many different roles that culminate in the final pathology report. Several software systems can be used to enhance/improve pathologist workflow. These systems include voice recognition software, pre–sign-out quality assurance, microscopic image embedding within surgical pathology reports, and computerized provider order entry. Recent changes in diagnostic coding and centralized electronic health records represent potential areas for increased ways to enhance/improve the workflow for surgical pathologists. Additional unforeseen changes to pathologist workflow may accompany the introduction of whole-slide imaging technology to the routine diagnostic work.

REFERENCES

1. Sarewitz SJ. Subspecialization in community pathology practice. Arch Pathol Lab Med 2014;138(7):871–2.
2. Black-Shaffer WS, Young RH, Harris NL. Subspecialization of surgical pathology at the Massachusetts General Hospital. Am J Clin Pathol 1996;106(4 Suppl 1): S33–42.
3. Groppi DE, Alexis CE, Sugrue CF, et al. Consolidation of the North Shore-LIJ Health System Anatomic Pathology Services: the challenge of subspecialization, operations, quality management, staffing and education. Am J Clin Pathol 2013; 140(1):20–30.

4. Henricks WH, Roumina K, Skilton BE, et al. The utility and cost effectiveness of voice recognition technology in surgical pathology. Mod Pathol 2002;15(5): 565–71.

5. Kang HP, Sirintrapun J, Nestler RJ, et al. Experience with voice recognition in surgical pathology at a Large Academic Multi-Institutional Center. Am J Clin Pathol 2010;133:156–9.

6. Singh M, Pal TR. Voice recognition technology implementation in surgical pathology. Arch Pathol Lab Med 2011;135:1476–81.

7. Serrano L, Hegge P, Sato B, et al. Using LEAN principles to improve quality, patient safety, and workflow in histology and anatomic pathology. Adv Anat Pathol 2010;17:215–21.

8. Zarbo RJ, Tuthill JM, D'Angelo R, et al. The Henry Ford Production System: reduction of surgical pathology in-process misidentification defects by bar code-specified work process standardization. Am J Clin Pathol 2009;131:468–77.

9. D'Angelo R, Zarbo RJ. The Henry Ford Production System: measures of process defects and waste in surgical pathology as a basis for quality improvement initiatives. Am J Clin Pathol 2007;128(3):423–9.

10. Zarbo RJ, D'Angelo R. The Henry Ford Production System: effective reduction of process defects and waste in surgical pathology. Am J Clin Pathol 2007;128(6): 1015–22.

11. Persoon TJ, Zaleski S, Frerichs J. Improving preanalytic processes using the principles of lean production (Toyota Production System). Am J Clin Pathol 2006;125(1):16–25.

12. Jimmerson C, Weber D, Sobek DK 2nd. Reducing waste and errors: piloting lean principles at Intermountain Healthcare. Jt Comm J Qual Patient Saf 2005;31(5): 249–57.

13. Grimm EE, Schmidt RA. Reengineered workflow in the anatomic pathology laboratory: costs and benefits. Arch Pathol Lab Med 2009;133:601–4.

14. Kohn LT, Corrigan JM, Donaldson MS, editors. To err is human: building a safer health system. Washington, DC: National Academy Press; 1999.

15. Nakhleh RE. What is quality in surgical pathology? J Clin Pathol 2006;59:669–72.

16. Owens SR, Dhir R, Yousem SA, et al. The development and testing of a laboratory information system-driven tool for pre-sign-out quality assurance of random surgical pathology reports. Am J Clin Pathol 2010;133:836–41.

17. Owens SR, Wiehagen LT, Kelly SM, et al. Initial experience with a novel pre-sign-out quality assurance tool for review of random surgical pathology diagnoses in a subspecialty-based University practice. Am J Surg Pathol 2010;34:1319–23.

18. Parwani AV, Mohanty SK, Becich MJ. Pathology reporting in the 21st century: the impact of synoptic reports and digital imaging. Lab Med 2008;39(10):582–6.

19. Leong AS. Synoptic/Checklist reporting of breast biopsies: has the time come? Breast J 2001;7:271–4.

20. Leong FJ, Leong AS. Digital imaging in pathology: theoretical and practical considerations, and applications. Pathology 2004;36:234–41.

21. Qu Z, Ninan S, Almosa A, et al. Synoptic reporting in tumor pathology: advantages of a web-based system. Am J Clin Pathol 2007;127:898–903.

22. Baskovich BW, Allan RW. Web-based synoptic reporting for cancer checklists. J Pathol Inform 2011;2:16.

23. Lankshear S, Srigley J, McGowan T, et al. Standardized synoptic cancer pathology reports – so what and who cares? A population-based satisfaction survey of 970 pathologists, surgeons, and oncologists. Arch Pathol Lab Med 2013;137(11): 1599–602.

24. Ellis DW. Surgical pathology reporting at the crossroads: beyond synoptic reporting. Pathology 2011;43(5):404–9.
25. Available at: http://www.ascp.org/PDF/Advocacy/Performance-Measures.pdf. Accessed August 29, 2014.
26. Devine EB, Hansen RN, Wilson-Norton JL, et al. The impact of computerized provider order entry on medication errors in a multispecialty group practice. J Am Med Inform Assoc 2010;17(1):78–84.
27. Baron JM, Dighe AS. Computerized provider order entry in the clinical laboratory. J Pathol Inform 2011;2:35.
28. Nakhleh RE, Gephardt G, Zarbo RJ. Necessity of clinical information in surgical pathology: a College of American Pathologists q-probes study of 771475 surgical pathology cases from 341 institutions. Arch Pathol Lab Med 1999;123:615–9.
29. Kinonen CL, Watkin WG, Gleason BC, et al. An audit of dermatopathology requisitions: hand written vs. electronic medical record data entry accuracy. J Cutan Pathol 2012;39:850–2.
30. Available at: http://en.wikipedia.org/wiki/A_picture_is_worth_a_thousand_words. Accessed August 30, 2014.
31. Appleton A, Sadek K, Dawson IG, et al. Clinicians were oblivious to incorrect logging of test dates and the associated risks in an online pathology application: a case study. Inform Prim Care 2012;20(4):241–7.
32. Nakhleh RE. Quality in surgical pathology communication and reporting. Arch Pathol Lab Med 2011;135:1394–7.
33. Available at: http://www.cms.gov/Medicare/Coding/ICD10/index.html?redirect=/icd10. Accessed August 30, 2014.

Specialized Laboratory Information Systems

Bryan Dangott, MD

KEYWORDS

• Specialty LIS • Report integration • Niche LIS • Multimodality LIS • Streamlined LIS
• Custom-build • Efficient LIS

OVERVIEW: WHAT IS A SPECIALIZED LABORATORY INFORMATION SYSTEM?

Broadly speaking, a specialized LIS is designed to perform a limited number of functions extremely well rather than trying to serve the needs of an entire laboratory. Because specialty systems are more customized than general LISs, they can take many forms. For example, a specialty LIS may exist as a stand-alone commercial application that is installed alongside an existing LIS architecture. Alternatively, they may consist of a markedly enhanced or customized spin-off or module of an existing LIS. Additionally, in practice settings where subspecialty sign-out is the norm, a specialty-specific LIS or LISs may fulfill all the needs of the organization. In rare instances, a specialty LIS may be developed entirely in-house to serve as the backbone of a laboratory. Some examples and characteristics of specialized LISs are listed in **Box 1**.

IDENTIFYING SHORTCOMINGS

Potential Shortcomings of an Existing Laboratory Information System

Some laboratories or laboratory sections have unique needs that traditional anatomic and clinical pathology systems may not address. Settings where a specialized LIS may thrive are listed in **Box 2**. The factors contributing to perceived or real shortcomings in a given laboratory with a given LIS are usually complicated and multifactorial. In most instances, laboratory sections do not have the luxury of choosing an LIS up front. More often than not, a laboratory with an existing LIS adapts its functions to the changing or growing role of the laboratory or laboratory subsections. Unfortunately, these adaptations may sometimes fall short of the desired outcome. Challenges for traditional LISs are listed in **Box 3**.

Potential Shortcoming of a New Laboratory Information System

When a laboratory is in the rare position of choosing a new LIS, the needs of the laboratory as a whole need to be considered in comparison to the needs of individual

This article originally appeared in Surgical Pathology Clinics, Volume 8, Issue 2, June 2015.
East Carolina University, 600 Moye Blvd, Greenville, NC 27834, USA
E-mail address: dangottb@ecu.edu

Clin Lab Med 36 (2016) 41–50
http://dx.doi.org/10.1016/j.cll.2015.09.005
labmed.theclinics.com

Box 1
General characteristics of a specialized laboratory information system

Performs a critical function
Example: interfaces with equipment that a traditional LIS does not support, allows future scalability

Enhances operations
Example: improved turnaround time, specimen tracking, enhanced reports, diagnostic data representation, correlation with previous results, etc.

Fills a major gap in existing systems
Example: allows meaningful and efficient storage and use of genomic or molecular testing, allows laboratories to adopt new testing methodologies

Tailored to specific practice environment
Example: subspecialty sign-out, molecular diagnostics, pharmaceutical industry

---

Box 2
Settings where a specialized laboratory information system may thrive

High-volume subspecialty sign-out
Example: dedicated sign-out of gastrointestinal, genitourinary, hematopathology, dermatopathology, etc.

Limited practice sign-out
Example: pharmaceutical or research setting, flow cytometry laboratory, molecular laboratory

Pathology practices trying to gain competitive advantage with enhanced functions
Example: customer relationship management, Web-based reports, integration of whole-slide images, molecular testing data, or photomicrographs with reports

Esoteric or cutting-edge testing
Example: transplant pathology, immunophenotyping, donor matching, flow cytometry, molecular testing, and proprietary testing methodologies, such as multigene tumor profiles, whole-slide imaging

High-throughput laboratories
Example: large commercial laboratory systems with LIS dashboards designed to track business and operational metrics and to streamline high-volume workflows

---

Box 3
Challenges for traditional laboratory information systems

Rapid growth of a laboratory section
Example: a previously considered low-priority feature may become critically important with laboratory growth

Evolving or proprietary test methodologies
Example: in-house developed test

New markets
Example: gene expression tumor profiling

New data types
Example: genomic sequencing

Integrated reports
Example: integration of histology, clinical laboratory data, flow cytometry, and molecular and cytogenetic testing methodologies as may be found in a hematopathology case

laboratory subsections. LIS purchase decisions are major financial investments with long-term contracts and significant organizational impact. The scale and complexity of these decisions may cause some unique or lower-priority requests to be outweighed by the operational needs of the laboratory or organization as a whole. The needs of every section in the laboratory often cannot be met by a single product. This may leave some laboratory sections with unmet needs. Furthermore, strong consideration should be given to the challenges of switching an LIS. Although technical barriers are in themselves difficult, an LIS conversion can be challenging from the perspectives of personnel and managing change within an organizational culture. The larger the organization, the greater the challenge in replacing a major component of an operational infrastructure.

Shortcomings due to Evolving Technology

Some clinical laboratory analyzers were originally designed for a research setting. These instruments may include their own software, which was designed to interact with the instrument. However, the software may not have well-developed options for interfacing with the traditional LIS or electronic medical (EMR) systems. These stand-alone systems may themselves be considered a specialty LIS. This is more common when a vendor focuses heavily on hardware, and, as a result, the software that accompanies the equipment may be underdeveloped. These systems can be harder to maintain and may require on-site experts to handle customization and technical support issues.

Shortcomings due to Nontraditional Data Sets

Laboratory testing is a rapidly evolving field with a significant number of new tests and techniques introduced every year. Gene sequencing and molecular testing can create massive data sets, which require customized storage and data processing solutions. A traditional LIS is not designed to handle these data sets. Even technologies, such as whole-slide imaging, can create a need for a specialty LIS. Most whole-slide imaging systems come with their own software, which in many cases fits the definition of a specialty LIS. In well-established laboratories, some modalities of testing may not even have existed when the original LIS was chosen, which can leave gaps in function for the LIS as other technologies mature.[1]

MEETING UNIQUE NEEDS

As discussed previously, there are many settings where a laboratory may have unique needs that are not addressed by the current LIS. If the needs for a laboratory are too unique, the market for software to address these needs may be small. Another laboratory that has similar needs may also have just enough differences in its requirements to make the design of a broadly marketable solution difficult. From a software design point of view, these site-to-site differences lead to market fragmentation. Large LIS vendors may avoid small niche markets for these exact reasons. Common features of a niche market are listed in **Box 4**. A specialty LIS vendor needs to generate enough revenue from a small customer base to overcome the high development costs. If demand or profitability is strong enough, a few vendors may be willing to take the risk of developing custom software.

Options for Filling Gaps

Option 1: Buying from an Existing Vendor
In many cases, LIS vendors offer add-on modules to augment their flagship systems. If an add-on exists that addresses an application gap, it should be strongly considered.

> **Box 4**
> **Features of a niche market**
>
> 1. Current products do not offer an adequate solution.
> 2. There is a motivated customer base with unmet needs.
> 3. Product development and marketing are tailored to a particular market segment.
> 4. Niche product offers better performance or unique attributes in comparison to other solutions.

Usually, a vendor-offered add-on can seamlessly integrate with existing infrastructure. The costs of implementing a vendor solution, however, can be too high if the specialty testing volume is low or if there are unknown/uncertain reimbursement streams. Rapidly evolving laboratory technologies are especially challenging because they may lack LIS vendor support initially. If the existing LIS vendor does not address the needs of a particular subsection, the laboratory could consider adding a specialty LIS to fill the gaps.

Option 2: Buying from a Separate Vendor
Some specialized LIS products comprise a self-contained LIS that exists in concert with an existing LIS. Adding infrastructure from a separate vendor raises considerable organizational costs in terms of licensing, personnel, and maintenance of multiple disparate systems. Balancing the complexity, efficiency, cost, technical support, and operational needs for these decisions is a challenge that is unique to every individual setting. For a laboratory purchasing a stand-alone LIS, this may translate to high up-front and long-term support costs. Some specialty LISs are hosted and supported off-site through cloud technologies that allow Web-based access and management. Off-site hosting may work well for some purposes, but there have to be clear Health Insurance Portability and Accountability Act protections in place and clear methods for archiving or exporting data if a vendor ever goes out of business. A special section is dedicated to discussing Web-based LIS reporting and off-site LISs later in this article.

Option 3: Bridging or Building
In some cases, buying a market ready product meets the needs of a laboratory. In other cases, alternative approaches to address the shortcomings are needed. For laboratories that are not satisfied with the existing market options, there are essentially 2 other approaches: bridge or build. These options can only be considered realistic if advanced technical skills are readily available within the organization. Building requires more technical expertise than bridging, but both approaches need an experienced information technology (IT) team.

Bridging Some vendors or in-house LIS teams are able to add functions to existing systems to enhance the performance of an LIS. For example, several anatomic LISs have macro or scripting languages or are built around word processing solutions, which have this capacity. Using these programming tools, menus and forms can be built to fill gaps in functionality. An advantage of this method is these changes can be made without major alteration in the LIS. The difficulty with this technique is maintaining consistency throughout all workstations because macro code is frequently deployed locally. Other solutions may be developed within an existing middleware product. However, as volumes increase, parent LISs are updated, or when new technologies are adopted, these bridge solutions may be overwhelmed or become outdated.

Building Some laboratories take greater ownership of the design and support of their LISs by designing their own modules or code where needed. Designing and implementing software to act as a specialized LIS requires significant planning, preparation, and training. Organizations that are considering this option usually undergo extensive evaluation of the initial and long-term economic implications of building their own systems.

Large-scale commercial laboratory Large-scale laboratories may think that available LIS products do not adequately meet all of their needs. In some exceptional settings, the right mix of technical staff, organizational need, and capital backing may exist to produce an entirely custom-built LIS product. A software system designed specifically for the needs of a laboratory not only can address shortcomings of other products but also can provide strategic advantages by addressing the specific needs of the organization, its workforce, and its customers. The up-front financial and time investments can be substantial, but the rewards come in the form of gained efficiencies and application flexibility. Considerations for building an in-house LIS are listed in **Box 5**. The long-term support of these products is usually performed in-house. In the right setting, the up-front costs may also be offset by lower long-term support and licensing fees.

CONSIDERATIONS FOR BUILDING AN IN-HOUSE LABORATORY INFORMATION SYSTEM MODULE

Scalability and Timeliness

Initially, an in-house LIS module may be developed to optimize a specific workflow. If a laboratory later decides to add additional testing modalities or workflows, a separate module may need to be built. This can be a slow development process and may delay a laboratory's entry into some testing markets. Many commercial LISs already have modules that may fit the general needs of the added modality. The implementation time for these new modules can, therefore, generally be done more quickly with a commercial product if one exists. If there is no acceptable product, then developing in house may be faster than waiting for a vendor solution.

Experience of the Design Team

The LIS is more than just a software product. It is a home to diagnostic patient information that has a critical function to the organizational mission. In addition, it is subject to extensive regulatory oversight by Clinical Laboratory Improvement Amendments and other accrediting agencies. The design team must be familiar with those constraints and also be able to work in concert with them. The design team needs to be staffed in such a way that the organization is protected from loss of one or several key personnel. A custom-built solution may be well understood by a few individuals. Retiring or departing staff who possess this intellectual capital can leave a knowledge

---

Box 5
Considerations for building an in-house laboratory information system

1. Scalability

2. Building a design team

3. Support costs

4. Total cost of ownership versus long-term benefit

gap that can be hard to fill. Extensive documentation and use of common coding languages and common backend architectures can be helpful in avoiding major knowledge gaps.

Support Costs

An in-house product has to factor in long-term maintenance costs before a project starts. An off-the-shelf LIS product usually comes with predictable maintenance costs. For sizable laboratories, the annual maintenance fees for a commercial LIS can exceed several hundred thousand dollars annually. Staff needs for developing a new system may far exceed the staff necessary to support the system. How to reallocate personnel on completion of the development phase of the project becomes a challenging question.

Cost Versus Benefit

The costs of implementation and support must be weighed in each setting to determine the best course of action. Some key questions to answer are

1. Will the system deliver strategic advantages to the laboratory?
2. Will the workflow be more efficient or allow more automation?
3. Will the in-house system allow customized reports that are strategically valuable to the client base?
4. Can integration with other systems and instrumentation be easily achieved?
5. Are Web-based reports a priority?
6. Are dollars that would be invested in LIS development better spent elsewhere?
7. What is the long-term impact of the LIS on the organization?
8. Does the in-house product allow better-quality management and improve operational efficiency?

NEWER TECHNOLOGIES AND REPORTING OPTIONS
The Off-Site LIS

Web-based LISs are relatively new and not widely implemented. The workflow of a Web-based LIS is well suited for integrated or enhanced result reporting. Several of the larger commercial laboratories have already implemented Web-based LISs for at least some of their workflow. In some respects, large commercial laboratories with Web portals act as specialized LISs for their clients. This is well suited for flow cytometry reporting, molecular reporting, cytogenetics, and esoteric testing. Web-based reporting may take on several forms depending on market conditions and client types. In a reference laboratory setting, the clientele may consist of hospitals, medical groups, individual physicians, or even individual patients. Web-based resulting offers the ability to download a fully graphical PDF report.[1,2] Clients may then use these graphical reports to show to patients.

There are some technical challenges of incorporating Web-based results with an existing LIS. First, a Web-based report may create a separate data stream which can present challenges for tracking the status of pending tests. Second, the results may be delivered in a format that is less conducive to integration with current systems. Many modern anatomic LISs have the capacity to archive an external document by attaching it to an existing accession number. This has big advantages for integrating various results and data sources with a case. Some LISs and EMRs allow importation of graphical elements via scanning, attaching an electronic file such as a PDF, or using Health Level Seven Clinical Document Architecture (CDA).[3]

Reporting Results to Clients

For Web-based resulting, the design of reporting groups is an important consideration. This is understood more clearly by considering that many individual users of a Web-based system may belong to the same client. Individual users may also share responsibility for patient results. Groups are created by allowing individual users to see results of other members in that group. Various levels of reporting groups are listed in **Box 6**. In general, more members in a reporting group may yield gains in convenience at the possible expense of security. No matter how the reporting groups are assigned, each user should always have a unique user name and password.

Example 1—Client Level Access

Consider that physicians 1, 2, 3, and 4 all work for Hospital ABC. A reference laboratory may wish to consider all the pathologists from Hospital ABC as a group. The individual users that are granted group level access may see results from all specimens sent in by any other user of that group. This setup helps with cross-coverage so that results for a case can be seen and acted on without delay if the original ordering pathologist is on vacation when the ancillary test results are delivered.

Example 2—Client Subgroups

In some settings, small groups of pathologists handle subspecialty sign-out for the practice. In sub-specialty diagnostic settings, physicians 1 and 2 may handle hematopathology results whereas physicians 3 and 4 handle dermatopathology testing. In this setting, it may be more beneficial to create client subgroups. This way the hematopathologists only have access to hematopathology testing data whereas the dermatopathologists only have access to dermatopathology data.

Example 3—Individual Access

Physician or individual level login is more limited and only allows given users to see results they have responsibility for on a given patient. Some direct-to-consumer laboratories use similar user level reporting so that patients may log in to see their own results through a portal.

Example 4—Result Level Reporting

Result level reporting means a unique login is created for each result. This is the most restrictive form of Web-based reporting. In this scenario, a unique login has to be

---

Box 6
Reporting groups

Client level
   Users in this group have access to all results for the client ID.

Group level
   Users in this group only have access to a specific reporting group. Individual users may belong to more than one group.

Individual level
   Individual users can only log in to see results from tests they are designated as responsible for. Individual level access may be for a physician or even a patient.

Result level
   Result level reporting means that each result is in its own group and the login only allows viewing of that specific test result.

delivered to the user for each result. If the credentials for viewing a Web-based result are delivered via reporting to a remote LIS, then the ability to track who has viewed the result is also lost because several users may view the log-in credentials, but it is not possible to track who actually logs in. When a user logs in, only the results from that specific test are viewable.[4]

EXAMPLE: HEMATOPATHOLOGY, THE SPECIALTY THAT CHALLENGES THE SPECIALIZED LABORATORY INFORMATION SYSTEM
Specialized Laboratories

Highly specialized laboratories that deal exclusively with specific specimen types occasionally have needs that can be better addressed by specialized LISs. Benefits may be gained in workflow solutions that are specifically tailored for the specimens and environment of the laboratory. Examples where this may occur include flow cytometry, hematopathology, gastrointestinal pathology, dermatopathology, and molecular testing. Of these, a hematopathology bone marrow specimen is a complex workflow that is good for illustrative purposes due to the amount of ancillary testing that may accompany a given specimen. Potential complexities of subspecialty testing are listed in **Box 7**.

Complex Workflow

Complex workflows may not be well addressed by traditional anatomic pathology LISs. Traditional anatomic pathology practice involves examining histologic sections in conjunction with appropriate use of immunohistochemical stains, special stains, in situ hybridization studies, and/or immunofluorescence studies. In general, these testing methods are available for interpretation within 1 day of being requested. A complete histologic interpretation for most surgical specimens is usually completed within a few days but same-day turnaround services exist.[5,6] The testing modalities of most surgical specimens are readily handled by a traditional anatomic LIS. Using the hematopathology bone marrow example (proposed previously), the complexity of data integration increases and reports can deviate significantly from traditional histopathology workflows.[7] With a bone marrow sample, the peripheral blood and bone marrow aspirate specimens may be morphologically evaluated on 1 day with a bone marrow core examined on day 2 after decalcification and paraffin embedding. Another day may pass while waiting for immunohistochemistry evaluation of the bone marrow core. If these specimens are triaged and dictated by a pathologist, this can involve multiple sessions of dictation, review, and editing before the slides are completely evaluated and a diagnostic report can be issued.

Box 7
Complexities of subspecialty testing

1. Complex workflow
2. Multimodality testing and data types
3. Varied reporting timeline
4. Integration of various data types and tests which may have their own reporting paradigm or be signed out at an off-site facility
5. Integration of various IT systems/varied control/ownership of testing modalities
6. Evolving technologies

Multimodality Testing and Data Types

Common testing methods that may challenge anatomic LISs include flow cytometry, diagnostic molecular studies, clonality studies, and cytogenetic studies. The usual turnaround times for some of the more complex ancillary testing methodologies can take days or weeks. This can present a problem for reporting these ancillary results when a diagnostic report has already been issued. The example bone marrow specimen frequently includes flow cytometry testing, fluorescence in situ hybridization (FISH) testing, cytogenetic testing, and/or various forms of molecular testing. The challenge for pathologists and LISs in general is integrating these varied testing methodologies and data types into a concise report. Flow cytometric, cytogenetic, and FISH reports may include images in addition to textual reports. Molecular testing may include graphs of historical values of transcript levels to show how a patient is responding to targeted agents.

Timeline

The third challenge in the hematopathology multimodality testing example is incorporating testing results into the diagnostic workflow with a timeline that is extended and unpredictable. Flow cytometry results are usually available in sync with the timeline of a primary bone marrow report. Cytogenetic results are usually not available before the bone marrow is ready for sign-out and must be added as an addendum. FISH and molecular testing have varied timelines but are generally available post–sign-out. Molecular clonality studies and esoteric gene profiling tests can take several weeks to perform. For pathologists, it may be difficult to keep track of where all specimens are in the testing timeline. A system that tracks pending tests and laboratory contact information can be helpful for updating the diagnostic report, for updating clinicians with findings of the ancillary studies, and for following up on "overdue" results. Most practices deal with these timeline incongruencies by adding addendums/amendments to the original histologic report to include ancillary testing results with a comment on the impact on the final diagnosis.

Data Integration from Multiple Laboratories

Another major challenge of specialty sign-out is that some testing may be performed off-site.[7] Off-site testing can get even more complex if a commercial laboratory triaged the specimen to multiple separate facilities. This adds complexity to both the uncertain timeline and interfacing issues (discussed previously). An ideal solution alerts a pathologist when a new result is available or automatically injects the data into a field on a pending amendment for later review. Automatic injection is only realistic for ancillary testing that is performed in the parent institution where contextual fields can be predefined and controlled. The structure of an ideal integrated report would approximately follow a synoptic template[8] to let clinicians know that some tests are still pending or that some tests were not performed. Design consistency helps clinicians find information quickly and provides a standardized structure where specific test results are expected to be found.[9] Using a well-structured report, the data from a particular testing methodology consistently fall in a specific location or under a specific header.

Multisystem

The fifth challenge of integration is crossing data between clinical pathology and anatomic pathology systems. If a laboratory has in-house testing, the results for FISH and molecular testing may be reported into the clinical pathology system. If testing is performed off-site, the results may or may not be interfaced to an existing clinical pathology system. If the systems are interfaced at all, they are most likely only transmitting textual data. Although technically possible, the probability of receiving graphical data over an interface at the present time is low. At the present time, integrating results from disparate systems into a single anatomic pathology report is generally done manually.

Evolving Technologies

As discussed previously, instrumentation and testing methodologies are rapidly evolving, which presents challenges to a traditional LIS. Hematopathology has a high adoption rate of new testing methodologies. Few LISs are designed to meet the data storage, integration, and reporting needs across anatomic pathology, flow cytometry, molecular, and cytogenetic modalities.

SUMMARY

This article examines the concepts underlying specialized LISs, their characteristics, and in what settings they may perform well. Opportunities for specialized LISs continue to evolve as whole-slide imaging, genetic testing, and personalized medicine efforts continue to grow.

REFERENCES

1. Park S, Pantanowitz L, Sharma G, et al. Anatomic pathology laboratory information systems: a reivew. Adv Anat Pathol 2012;19(2):81–96.
2. Winsten D. The Web-enabled LIS. Advance for the Laboratory 2005;14:9 38.
3. Dolin R, Alschuler L, Boyer S, et al. HL7 clinical document architecture, release 2. J Am Med Inform Assoc 2006;13:30–9.
4. Shirts B, Larsen N, Jackson B. Utilization and utility of clinical laboratory reports with graphical elements. J Pathol Inform 2012;3:26.
5. López A, Graham A, Barker G, et al. Virtual slide telepathology enables an innovative telehealth rapid breast care clinic. Hum Pathol 2009;40:1082–91.
6. Barentsz M, Wessels H, van Diest P, et al. Same-day diagnosis based on histology for women suspected of breast cancer: high diagnostic accuracy and favorable impact on the patient. PLoS One 2014;9(7):1–6.
7. Hess J. What hematopathology tells us about the future of pathology informatics. Arch Pathol Lab Med 2009;133:908–11.
8. Mohanty S, Piccoli A, Devine L, et al. Synoptic tool for reporting of hematological and lymphoid neoplasms based on World Health Organization classification and College of American Pathologists checklist. BMC Cancer 2007;7:144.
9. Valenstein P. Formatting pathology reports: applying four design principles to improve communication and patient safety. Arch Pathol Lab Med 2008;132:84–94.

Laboratory Information Systems Management and Operations

Ioan C. Cucoranu, MD

KEYWORDS

- LIS management • LIS operations • Change control • End-user training
- Quality control reports • Help desk

OVERVIEW

The main mission of an LIS is to manage a laboratory's workflow (both specimens and patient data) and to deliver accurate results for clinical management, in a timely manner. A modern LIS should have built-in functionality for other required activities, such as regulations, billing, or quality assurance. Currently, in the United States, pathology laboratories are under continuous pressure to improve workflows by using lean initiatives. Technologies, such as tracking systems and automation, have been used successfully for decades in clinical laboratories; they are finally becoming the norm in pathology laboratories as well. Other useful LIS functions, particularly when used in an academic environment, are support for pathology education and research.

The successful selection and implementation of an anatomic pathology LIS is not complete unless it is complemented by long-term specialized information technology (IT) support. This should be provided by both in-house informatics and IT resources as well as by an LIS vendor. Nevertheless, optimal LIS operations depend on the availability of adequate, dedicated, and skilled informatics and IT personnel. For large health care systems, collaboration and communication between a laboratory's LIS staff and the hospital-wide IT personnel play a key role in the successful LIS maintenance.[1]

A LIS is required to remain continuously operational with minimal or no downtime. At the same time, an LIS team has to ensure that all operations are compliant with the mandated rules and regulations. As is the case for any health information system (HIS), close attention should also be shown to a system's development life cycle to further improve its functionality and usability. **Box 1** lists key operations that any LIS team needs to handle post–system implementation.

This article originally appeared in Surgical Pathology Clinics, Volume 8, Issue 2, June 2015.
Department of Pathology and Laboratory Medicine, University of Florida College of Medicine - Jacksonville, 655 West 8th Street, Room 1-078, Jacksonville, FL 32209-6596, USA
E-mail address: ioan.cucoranu@jax.ufl.edu

Box 1
Key operations that laboratory information system teams need to handle post–system implementation

- Training
- Help desk support
- Change control
- System security
- System data backup
- Interface monitoring and maintenance
- Downtime management (unscheduled vs scheduled)
- Database maintenance
- Upgrades (software and hardware)
- Administrative and management reporting
- Budgeting and cost analysis
- System validation
- Documentation
- New product evaluation
- Quality assurance and quality improvement initiatives

SYSTEM VALIDATION

Although a tedious and costly process, LIS validation must be performed to prove that an implemented system is fit for its intended use and that the system manages information well, with the expected accuracy, reliability, and file integrity, both initially and over time.[2] During the validation process, various LIS functions are performed while data are collected, maintained, and independently reviewed to demonstrate that the system performs consistently according to specifications. Pathology laboratories must establish protocols and standards for the validation process. All the validation steps and results must be well documented.

LIS vendors perform initial, internal system validations; however, any system must be revalidated whenever end users, vendors, or third parties add modifications or customizations. The Clinical and Laboratory Standards Institute published important factors that should be considered when developing validation protocols for LISs, including recommendations for preparation of validation protocols, to assess the accuracy and dependability of LISs in storing, retrieving, and transmitting data.[3]

INTERFACE MAINTENANCE AND MONITORING

Electronic interfaces are critical components of any HIS, having a significant impact on the overall performance of information exchange and health care delivery. They allow transmission of data and information between LISs and other clinical information systems (eg, electronic medical records and billing systems) or between LISs and laboratory equipment (eg, automated immunohistochemistry slide stainers). Although electronic interfaces have been in use for years and attempts have been made to standardize their implementation, the whole process is still a time- and resource-consuming process. Interface customization depends significantly on the laboratory and clinical systems being connected and on how those systems have been implemented.

Once implemented, additional activities are necessary to monitor and maintain interfaces, especially whenever changes are performed on any of the systems involved. Pathology laboratories are responsible for identifying interface problems (eg, laboratory orders not being processed or report formatting issues). Laboratory directors must ensure the outcomes of critical LIS functionality.[4] These include

- Accurate and complete flow of information between LISs and electronic health records
- Logical and human-readable report formatting on the receiving end and maintaining the essential elements of reports, as they were entered into the LIS
- Appropriate transmission of any coded information used to correctly identify results, such as LOINC
- Appropriate handling of report versioning, comments, or abnormality flags

Software packages to automate interface testing and validation are currently available. Keystrokes or data entry can be simulated and screen output reading can be performed electronically, to verify achievement of the desired outcomes. There are several advantages when using validation software tools, including the following:

- Scenarios can be checked multiple times.
- Outputs may be rigorously compared against intended outcomes.
- All interactions can be audited.
- A complete set of testing can be easily run whenever an adjustment is made to any system.

Key points to consider when maintaining and validating interfaces:

- Design a standardized process for recurrent interface validation.
- Perform the test on the entire chain of interfaces.
- Ensure that interface error logs work as expected and that there is a monitoring procedure in place.
- Use a test environment whenever possible.
- Use test patients when working in a live environment.
- Consider automated testing software to make the testing process faster, more accurate, more complete, reproducible, and better documented.
- Have a written agreement with the management of any receiving system, acknowledging the responsibility to inform the laboratory of any significant changes (eg, upgrades) so that timely revalidation can be performed.

TRAINING

End-user training is a critical component for a successful HIS implementation. Training components include

- Initial trainin—training administered to all users immediately before implementation of a brand-new LIS as well as training administered to newly hired staff
- Additional training—sessions provided to end users as their role and activities performed are changed or as additional features are added to the LIS.

For an effective training program development, it is important to assess end users' training needs by using techniques that reveal end users' cognitive processes. Usability testing methods have the ability to gather data related to human computer interaction.[5] These methods can be combined with traditional methods, such as interviews and questionnaire surveys.

HELP DESK SUPPORT

It is essential to implement well-planned support processes and procedures to minimize end-user frustration. The support system outcome could ultimately have a direct impact on LIS functionality. Help desk is a resource made available to end users when they encounter problems with their LIS services. Usually, the LIS help desk support specialists provide technical assistance with personal computers, operating systems, and LIS-related applications (eg, password log-ins and word processors) and sometimes with peripheral devices (eg, digital cameras) or add-on software (eg, voice recognition software) used in the laboratory. Help desk personnel may provide ad hoc end-user training on the proper use of all these components. Based on laboratory size and the help desk request volume, software applications can be implemented to support this process.

Implementation of best practices for help desk support include

- Knowledge management—system that improves operational efficiencies by reducing the time spent to rediscover previous incidents or problems
- Problem management—system that gathers information during incident management to help identify problems. Thus, the root cause of frequent recurring incidents can be identified by capturing information in a knowledge database.
- Access management—maintains end-user accounts along with password resets to ensure quick response time

CHANGE CONTROL AND DOCUMENTATION

Once an LIS is implemented, additional changes may be required by the vendor, IT services, or laboratory (eg, fine-tune, add functionality or add additional tests and protocols). Change control is a systematic approach used to manage all the changes made to an LIS. This approach ensures that no unnecessary or unauthorized changes are made, that all changes are documented and monitored in a controlled and coordinated fashion, that LIS services are not unnecessarily disrupted, and that laboratory IT and informatics resources are used efficiently. Planning, policies, and standard operation procedures (SOPs) as well as adherence to change control processes can potentially prevent a laboratory from costly mistakes (eg, system crashes, security breaches, or data corruption). Change control applies to any changes (eg, revisions, alterations, additions, enhancements, or upgrades) performed on both hardware and software. Furthermore, regulatory bodies, such as the College of American Pathologists, mandate documentation of all changes. LIS managers are responsible for change control documentation. **Table 1** lists recommended items to be documented as part of change control.

MANAGEMENT REPORTING AND QUALITY ASSURANCE/QUALITY IMPROVEMENT INITIATIVES

A modern LIS should be capable of generating automated or on-demand management reports, such as documentation for regulatory compliance, quality assurance, or monitoring performance and productivity (eg, turnaround time, abnormal results, reimbursement, or frozen section correlations). The LIS team should work closely with laboratory administration and the quality assurance team to create and generate the reports needed. If deemed necessary and cost effective, additional tolls could be

Table 1 Change control documentation	
Documentation Items	**Explanation of Change**
Description of change	Detailed explanation of the change performed
Reason for change	Needs and benefits of the performed change
Persons responsible for change implementation	Allow for identification of personnel that actually performed the change
Change category	Hardware, software, process, or procedural
Degree of change	Minor vs major—based on overall impact on the LIS, health care IT system, and laboratory, including cost
Change sign off	Identifies the person responsible for the overall change
Risk assessment	Allows for problems that may occur as result of the change to be assessed and planning for resolution if such problems occur
Evaluation and monitoring of the implemented changes	Evaluate outcome and determine the success of change implementation

Adapted from Cucoranu I, Parwani A, Pantanowitz L. Laboratory information system operations and regulations. In: Pantanowitz L, Parwani AV, editors. Practical informatics for cytopathology, vol. 14. New York: Springer; 2014. p. 64; with permission.

developed and/or implemented either in collaboration with an LIS vendor (vendor-assisted software modifications) or by using third-party middleware software packages.[6] A further detailed description of the informatics role in patient safety and quality assurance is provided in the article elsewhere in this issue.

DATABASE MAINTENANCE

Accurate and reliable data are integral to all the pathology laboratory processes that involve the use of LISs. Increased data processing and electronic data exchange heavily rely on accurate, reliable, controllable, and verifiable data recorded in databases. Data dictionaries are used to ensure data accuracy and standardization. LIS database dictionaries are dynamic documents that must be updated as data collection requirements change. Procedures should be in place to standardize database dictionaries maintenance.

NEW PRODUCT EVALUATION

Modern LISs in pathology laboratories provide an opportunity for implementation of data automation. Therefore, it is desirable when selecting, purchasing, and implementing new equipment in a laboratory to have the LIS team actively involved in evaluating the possibility and cost-effectiveness of data transfer via electronic interfaces. Similarly, when implementing digital imaging equipment, the LIS team should be involved in assessing digital imaging format compatibility with the current LIS.

Other LIS operations include LIS data security, reliability, and privacy of patient health information. These are important functions for any pathology laboratory; therefore, they are discussed in detail in a separate article.

REFERENCES

1. Cucoranu I, Parwani A, Pantanowitz L. Laboratory information system operations and regulations. In: Pantanowitz L, Parwani AV, editors. Practical informatics for cytopathology, vol. 14. New York: Springer; 2014. p. 61–70.

2. Cowan DF, Gray RZ, Campbell B. Validation of the laboratory information system. Arch Pathol Lab Med 1998;122:239–44.
3. Pearson S, Fuller J, Kowalski B, et al. Managing and validating laboratory information systems; Approved Guideline AUT08-A. 2007. 26. Available at: http://www.clsi.org/source/orders/free/AUT08-A.pdf. Accessed August 31, 2014.
4. Beckwith BA, Brassel JH, Brodsky VB, et al. Laboratory interoperability best practices: ten mistakes to avoid. College of American Pathologists; 2013. Available at: http://www.cap.org/apps/docs/committees/informatics/cap_dihit_lab_interop_final_march_2013.pdf. Accessed August 31, 2014.
5. Qiu Y, Yu P, Hyland P. A multi-method approach to assessing health information systems end users' training needs. Stud Health Technol Inform 2007;129:1352–6.
6. Kamat S, Parwani AV, Khalbuss WE, et al. Use of a laboratory information system driven tool for pre-signout quality assurance of random cytopathology reports. J Pathol Inform 2011;2:42.

Molecular Pathology Informatics

Somak Roy, MD

KEYWORDS

- Molecular informatics ● Next-generation sequencing ● Clinical informatics
- Bioinformatics

OVERVIEW

Molecular pathology has emerged as a major arsenal for promoting and sustaining personalized health care in modern medicine. In contrast to other ancillary diagnostic tools, molecular pathology delivers a wide spectrum of theranostic information starting from as little as a minute fragment of tissue or a simple blood draw. The results of molecular testing are significantly more complex than a simple numerical value or a binary outcome (yes/no). The post–Human Genome Project era has witnessed the most significant developments in genomics that has impacted the way clinical medicine is practiced today. Personalized medicine, which enables patient-specific therapeutic and disease management protocols, is being increasingly boosted and supported by the results of molecular testing performed on tissue biopsies and resections. In addition, it also serves as a valuable diagnostic tool in morphologically challenging cases. Genomic profiling of certain cancers, such as lung, colon, and melanoma, are now considered to be the standard of care for guiding appropriate treatment protocols. Very recently, a global molecular testing guideline was published for molecular testing of lung cancers by the collaborative efforts of College of American Pathologists, International Association for the Study of Lung Cancer, and Association for Molecular Pathology.[1] The Cancer Genome Atlas project (http://cancergenome.nih.gov/) over the past few years has released a wealth of genomic profiling information about major tumor types that had significantly fueled the discovery of potential actionable biomarkers for routine clinical use.[2-8]

A wide array of assay methodologies and platforms are used in laboratories for performing molecular testing, such as Sanger sequencing, real-time polymerase chain reaction (PCR), allele-specific PCR, DNA and RNA in situ hybridization (ISH), multiplex ligation-dependent probe amplification, microarray technology, and, more recently, next-generation sequencing (NGS) technology. The choice of platform depends on the question(s) answered by the clinical test and its appropriate applicability to patient care.

This article originally appeared in Surgical Pathology Clinics, Volume 8, Issue 2, June 2015.
Department of Pathology, Molecular and Genomic Pathology, University of Pittsburgh Medical Center, 3477 Euler way, Pittsburgh, PA 15213, USA
E-mail address: roys@upmc.edu

MOLECULAR INFORMATICS

Given the increasing popularity and relevance of high-complexity molecular testing in surgical pathology, where does informatics fit into the equation? To answer this question, it is important to understand the major operational domains of informatics, namely bioinformatics (BI) and clinical informatics (CI). Bioinformatics is a dynamic and rapidly evolving multidisciplinary field of informatics that has emerged out of the application of computational, mathematical, and statistical methods to investigate biological phenomena. BI dates back to as early as the 1960s, when fundamental discoveries in molecular biology were made. With more recent data deluge and development of massive repositories of biological and genomic data, the symbiotic relationship between molecular biology and BI has fueled mutual exponential growth.[9–11] Large and complex data (so-called big data), data-driven analytics, statistical modeling, development of new algorithms, and discovering meaningful and relevant information from raw biological data is inherent to BI.[10] In contrast, CI is a more established discipline that has developed and matured over a longer period of time with rigorous testing and validation in a clinical environment. CI implementations in health care systems are typically on an enterprise scale, using industry standard software and hardware with principal focus on secure and reliable data transmission, storage, retrieval, and interoperability between information systems and wide variety of medical devices rather than data-driven analytics and discovery. One of the key differences between BI and CI is application development environment and life cycle, which gives rise to several other differences between the two disciplines. Application development in BI is centered on a fundamental genomic or biological phenomenon that is under investigation in a given research project. The pace of design, testing, implementation, and troubleshooting (software patches) is typically coupled with the progress of the research project. If a BI application is successful and is usable across a wider user community, further improvement and maintenance is supported by open-source software development. The overall life cycle is fast paced but with variable support, documentation, and version control. CI applications (such as electronic medical record [EMR], laboratory information system [LIS]), in contrast, have a much tighter and longer development and implementation life cycle. Vendors usually provide formal application support, tight version control, and extensive documentation. Updates for feature enhancements and patches for troubleshooting are relatively infrequent and often expensive.

This conceptual distinction has existed for several years in clinical laboratories with minimal interactions between the two disciplines. With conventional molecular testing instrumentation, vendors were able to mask the complexity of underlying BI with a point-and-click user interface. However, with the speedy introduction of NGS testing in clinical laboratories, molecular pathology has finally broken this barrier, forming a unique collaborative environment for development of informatics solutions that bridge the gap between BI and CI. The term molecular informatics (MI) is often loosely used to refer to various informatics principles and operations in a molecular laboratory. The rapid advance in this domain during a short period of time has manifested its presence in the practice of molecular pathology.

Conceptually, MI forms the core conduit for generating, processing, porting, and management of the molecular data points from each step of every assay performed in the molecular laboratory. With increasing sophistication of the assay platform and workflow elements, the magnitude and complexity of the generated information increases exponentially. Surprisingly, MI has largely been an unrealized and neglected part of laboratory workflow, until the introduction of NGS technology in clinical laboratories.

Even a basic quantitative PCR instrument performs significant computation for generating and displaying results that the user is typically unaware of. The practice of conventional molecular laboratories has been centered on paper-based manual data management for targeted analysis and low complexity testing for several years. However, the colossal data surge as a result of NGS based testing breaks the capacity of this conventional system. As a consequence, the critical role of MI has been realized on a global scale, initiating several large-scale efforts across different organizations to develop principles and guidelines for developing information systems that can appropriately manage, present, and share molecular data.[12–15] Although MI encompasses a wide range of functions across the entire workflow for different testing platforms in the molecular laboratory, because of the limited scope of this article, only a broad overview of the different aspects of MI that pertains mostly to NGS testing is presented to the readers, given its significant impact and clinical relevance.

NEXT-GENERATION SEQUENCING

After the invention of Sanger sequencing in 1977[16] and PCR in 1985,[17] several important technological developments were witnessed that improved the practice of molecular pathology significantly. However, NGS has been a revolutionary change that has not only transformed the concepts and practice of molecular pathology testing but also affected the paradigm of disease management in clinical medicine and oncology. NGS enables very large-scale measurements of the genome, yielding an unprecedented amount of potentially valuable information.[18] This is unlike any other conventional molecular testing technology that has been in existence. For example, to perform a complete molecular profiling of a lung adenocarcinoma using conventional methods, DNA sequence variations (mutations) are detected using Sanger sequencing, real-time PCR, and other modalities. Gene fusions and copy number changes are detected using ISH technologies. Gene expression, if indicated, is typically detected using reverse-transcriptase PCR coupled with quantitative real-time PCR. Information on gene methylation, such as *MGMT* and *MLH1*, is obtained by methylation-specific PCR. In contrast, all of this testing can be performed using NGS on a single platform.

NGS testing can not only to detect sequence variations, but also gene fusions, copy number changes, gene expression, methylation profile, and large structural alterations from a single run on a single platform, making it a very efficient technology in clinical medicine. The high capacity of NGS sequencers allows multiplexing of several patient samples on a single run in a cost-effective way using DNA barcodes.[13,19] The underlying massively parallel sequencing of millions to billions of DNA fragments and subsequent preservation of information on every individual sequencing reads leverages extracting such a wide repertoire of genomic information.[18] The sequence reads can be manipulated and measured using diverse algorithms to derive the appropriate information.

Not surprisingly therefore, the scope for clinical application of NGS testing is expansive to include pharmacogenomics, somatic tumor profiling, minimal residual disease monitoring, and inherited diseases testing. Clinical NGS testing has been most applicable (and somewhat economically viable) to somatic profiling of solid and hematologic tumors using targeted resequencing of regions or genes of interest.[20–23] NGS-based molecular testing in surgical pathology has unraveled the next level of diagnostic and therapeutic stratification that is highly relevant for targeted therapy, subsequent management, and follow-up of patients. Cytology and tissue biopsies are a critical triage point for rendering an immediate diagnosis and subsequent submission of appropriate tissue for molecular testing.

NEXT-GENERATION SEQUENCING INFORMATICS

As mentioned briefly in the preceding section, discrete preservation of sequencing reads is a critical aspect of NGS technology that leverages a wealth of information about the interrogated genome. NGS data processing involves several sequential steps that are performed by different software applications in tandem, which is commonly referred to as a "pipeline." **Fig. 1** illustrates a simplified version of an NGS pipeline. Depending on the NGS platform used, the raw sequencing data are represented as a high-definition image file or as electrical signal trace with embedded features.[18] This information is unusable for detecting abnormalities in the genome as is, and therefore requires further processing to generate sequence information in a more appropriate format for consumption by downstream processes. This is also referred to as primary data processing and involves signal processing to generate raw sequence reads and subsequent alignment to the reference genome. An important feature to note is the magnitude and complexity of the data generated by a typical NGS instrument. The size of an individual sequencing file is roughly proportional to the number of sequencing reads contained in them and range in size from approximately 0.2 GB to 200 GB, depending on the scope of genomic measurements performed. During a pipeline execution, several intermediate files of significant magnitude also are generated that contribute to the total bulk of NGS data. The standard processes in an analytical pipeline, such as sequence alignment and variant detection on aligned sequence reads, are resource hungry. Multiple CPU cores and large amounts of Random Access Memory in a high-performance desktop workstation or a compute cluster environment are prerequisites. In terms of software, most of these analytical pipelines are optimized to run on a Unix or Linux operating system (OS).[24]

Subsequent to the primary data analysis of NGS data, secondary and tertiary downstream analyses are essential components of the global analytical pipeline in a clinical laboratory environment. The secondary analysis involves detection of variants (genomic alterations) using different algorithms (see **Fig. 1**). Tertiary analyses involve variant annotation, filtering, prioritization, variant and other public database lookups, data visualization tools, literature review, and knowledge-based management. These analytical steps can be performed by a combination of a wide variety of software, many of which are in active development and require constant support and improvement by the developer.[24] From a laboratory management standpoint, it is critical to understand the need for validating software pipelines in general to ensure highly accurate and reliable molecular test results due to their significant impact on therapeutic management.[12]

BIG DATA AND CLOUD COMPUTING

With increasing use of NGS and constant improvement in software algorithms, data processing and generation is voluminous but faster and more productive. This has led to rapid accumulation of datasets that are of astronomical scale (typically several terabytes to petabytes) that defy the conventional computational capacity for processing and storage. Data with this property is commonly referred to as big data. The concept of big data is relatively recent and there exists no widely accepted threshold or definition, as "big" is quite relative. The National Institute of Standards and Technology and other major enterprises, such as Google, Oracle, and Microsoft, have proposed their own definitions of big data.[25] Terabytes of data may not be "big" for an organization with access to enterprise data centers or a cloud computing environment, but may be "big" for organizations with a small to medium-scale information technology (IT) infrastructure. Big data existed in health care systems even before its

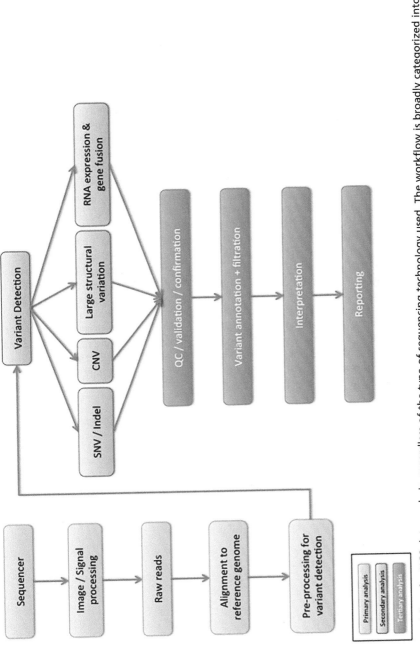

Fig. 1. A simplified workflow for NGS data analysis, regardless of the type of sequencing technology used. The workflow is broadly categorized into primary (*orange*), secondary (*purple*), and tertiary (*blue*) analysis steps. A wide repertoire of software applications can perform the individual steps in the workflow. It is important to note that for accuracy of clinical test results, each of the components of the analytical pipeline should be appropriately optimized and validated. CNV, copy number variation; QC, quality control; SNV, single nucleotide variant.

true realization in the post-genome era. Rapid introduction of NGS testing has led to confrontation with many challenges in implementation, but in parallel has also initiated innovation on a global scale to improve health care IT infrastructure to support genomics-driven personalized health care.[26,27] The 4 V's that define the elements of big data from a digital marketing perspective are velocity, volume, variety, and veracity.[28] NGS testing generates large amounts of data in a short period of time that contains a wide variety of information, which is often unpredictable at the initiation of testing and therefore confirms to the 4 elements of big data. Handling "big" genomic data and integrating with clinical data points in LISs and EMRs is an enormous task that will require significant collaboration among various stakeholders in health care.[26,28] The benefit of big data analytics is the power to predict clinical outcomes based on insight into archived clinical data in LISs and EMRs.[26] As NGS testing continues in health care, archived data will be enriched with genomic information, which when subjected to big data analytics will reveal potentially highly relevant information for cost-effective clinical decision-making. Such data-driven clinical decision support systems are under active research and development.

Intertwined with big data analytics is the concept of cloud computing. Cloud computing hosts a wide variety of functions, which are rendered as services to consumers for storing and processing data. Because hardware and software infrastructure is instantly scalable (up or down) based on the needs of the end user, it is a valuable and cost-effective resource for storing large data sets and performing complex data analysis. Cloud computing provides an ideal environment for data analytical requirements for NGS testing.[29–31] Laboratories do not require large capital investment on setting up and maintaining hardware and software infrastructure and still reap the benefits at a relatively low cost. Maintenance functions, such as data backup, redundancy generation, data security, and troubleshooting without downtime, are typically inclusive in the subscription fee.[31]

INFORMATICS CHALLENGES FOR NEXT-GENERATION SEQUENCING–BASED CLINICAL TESTING

Despite the various advantages of NGS testing, big data and cloud computing in molecular pathology, the real-world implementation of NGS poses several informatics challenges and concerns. The principal bottlenecks are centered on genomic data management, data security, and systems interoperability. There may be additional informatics challenges that are specific to an organization's local circumstances and therefore not included in this discussion.

Data Storage

NGS instruments generate a tremendous volume of data per sample per run. The magnitude scales are proportional to the scope of genomic measurements (targeted sequencing, whole exome, whole genome).[18] Data storage in external hard disk drives is not practical or reliable. It is recommended that clinical genomic data be backed up automatically into a secure off-site storage facility (such a disaster recovery center) with enough redundancy to allow minimum downtime for data recovery after a catastrophic event. Data storage should also allow use of alternate analytical pipelines on the archived data for validation and development. Thankfully, the cost per MB of data has dramatically decreased to sustain increasing storage requirements.[31] However, the initial capital investment to set up or use large-scale data backup facilities may be prohibitive depending on the institution's existing IT infrastructure. Given the increasing adaptation of high-throughput sequencing platforms in clinical laboratories, appropriate forecasting and budgeting of computing resource requirements is critical to avoid unexpected downtime in clinical testing. Unplanned data management also may increase the cost of storage (eg, storing raw sequencing data indefinitely). It is therefore important for molecular laboratories to set up reasonable retention policies for high-volume data. Unfortunately, there are no recommendations or guidelines available as of date that can be used by clinical laboratories, which adds to the complexity for forecasting resources.

Networking Infrastructure

One of the critical elements of handling NGS data, that is often overlooked until confronted with, is appropriate network connectivity for moving NGS datasets. It is an integral component of data archiving, data sharing across multiple users, and reusing the primary data for alternative analysis. A typical 10/100 Mbps local area network infrastructure that exists by default in most institutions cannot support the movement of massive NGS datasets and often affects other critical network-dependent hospital operations, such as EMR and LIS transactions. It is therefore imperative to include appropriate network requirements as part of the discussion with the IT team when implementing NGS in clinical laboratories.

Computing Infrastructure

As described previously, NGS data processing is resource intensive. That being said, the actual requirements are highly variable depending on the sequencing platform used and the scope of measurements desired. Constant improvements in algorithms for NGS data processing have allowed optimized use of memory and CPU cores allowing high-throughput analysis on desktop workstations. Although such a setup is not ideal in a production (clinical) environment for several reasons, including limited room for scaling up, it is often the most immediately practical and affordable solution. More appropriate and long-term solutions require setting up high-performance compute cluster or distributed compute grid with the flexibility of scaling up or down based on the laboratory's requirement.[28,31] This however requires technical expertise, involvement of the institution's IT group, and significant capital investment. The final decision for a given institution requires striking a balance and involvement of a multidisciplinary team of molecular pathologists, pathology informatics, bioinformaticians, and clinical IT personnel.

Data Security

Cloud computing provides the "next-generation" environment for cost-effective data analytics and management. Cloud computing environments are broadly classified into private (institutional), public, and hybrid depending on the access profile and relationship to an institution's firewall.[28,32] Public clouds are maintained by large commercial companies, which offer a wide variety of computing services without significant upfront capital investment. However, the principal concern in use of public clouds for health care data is data privacy and compliance with appropriate federal and institutional regulation.[32] Breach of hospital-managed clinical data is detrimental to its clients (patients), as well as the reputation of the institution itself. The clinical laboratory community with the current state of cloud computing is hesitant to use such services, despite all the technical and economic advantages. This is a domain of active development and there is drive toward appropriate auditing of public cloud services to ensure compliance with health care data privacy laws, albeit with the possibility of increase in associated cost of such services.[32]

Institutional cloud (private) setup is more attractive from a clinical laboratory perspective because it provides all the advantages of cloud computing but in a highly secure environment where the clinical data stays behind the firewall. The major limitation in implementing a private cloud is the significant capital, manpower, and infrastructure investment that may not be practical for many if not all organizations.

Privacy concerns surrounding genomic data in health care have been a matter of active discussion and fueled more recently by clinical NGS testing. The Health Insurance Portability and Accountability Act (HIPAA), enacted in 1996, enforces the adoption of privacy protection modalities by the federal government across all entities that hold protected health information (PHI).[33] There has been subsequent modification to HIPAA and enactment of additional laws (HITECH, 2009) and the Patient Protection and Affordable Care Act (ACA, 2010) to strengthen PHI security. With the adoption of new rules for privacy, security, and breach notification, in the final "HIPAA Omnibus Rule" (2013), genomic information has been designated as PHI.[34] This significantly impacts the storage and management of large-scale genomic information in clinical laboratories, including options for using cloud-based services.

Interoperability

A typical molecular pathology laboratory houses different analytical instruments that generate data and require some form of integration with existing informatics resource pool within the laboratory (custom database, Excel spreadsheets, LIS, shared pool for data storage). Unlike conventional molecular analytical instruments, NGS instruments allow network connectivity for bidirectional data transfer and sequence data archiving. However, NGS instruments by default do not support messaging protocols to interoperate between other CI systems or software. Additionally, significant technical challenges arise when interoperating NGS instruments that run on a UNIX-based OS with a hospital informatics infrastructure that typically runs on a Windows-based OS. IT support for a UNIX-based system may often be a significant bottleneck in deploying and maintaining NGS instruments. This necessitates development of middleware solutions to optimize NGS operations. Due to the substantial learning curve associated with establishing common grounds with the 2 disciplines, it is critical for molecular laboratories to involve bioinformaticians in active clinical NGS operations to foster collaborative development with CI.

Downstream (tertiary) NGS data analytics pose additional interoperability challenges. There are several applications (freeware, proprietary and custom developed) that are available or are in constant development to facilitate downstream data analysis, including interoperability with existing clinical systems using standard messaging protocols.

FUTURE PERSPECTIVE

Massively parallel sequencing technology has significantly impacted the traditional practice of clinical medicine and has led to a paradigm change in diagnostic and therapeutic principles of various diseases. Despite the promising outcomes of using NGS-based clinical testing, some of the critical bottlenecks (described previously), as well as the general constraining economic and regulatory environment, threatens full-scale implementation in clinical laboratories. Implementing NGS assays not only requires capital investment for purchase of appropriate hardware and reagents but also demands significant investment in acquiring skilled technical personnel, bioinformaticians, full-time employees for managing billing and customer service relationships, and a strong informatics infrastructure that is flexible enough to scale on demand and bridge the gap between BI and CI and support laboratory operations. Interestingly enough, despite these perplexing challenges, there is an increasing trend in adopting NGS testing across clinical laboratories. As NGS technology is maturing in the clinical domain, MI is going to play a key role in setting a stable ground.

REFERENCES

1. Lindeman NI, Cagle PT, Beasley MB, et al. Molecular testing guideline for selection of lung cancer patients for EGFR and ALK tyrosine kinase inhibitors: guideline from the College of American Pathologists, International Association for the Study of Lung Cancer, and Association for Molecular Pathology. J Mol Diagn 2013;15:415–53.
2. Cancer Genome Atlas Research Network. Comprehensive molecular profiling of lung adenocarcinoma. Nature 2014;511:543–50.
3. Cancer Genome Atlas Research Network. Comprehensive molecular characterization of gastric adenocarcinoma. Nature 2014;513:202–9.
4. Cancer Genome Atlas Research Network. Comprehensive molecular characterization of urothelial bladder carcinoma. Nature 2014;507:315–22.
5. Cancer Genome Atlas Research Network, Kandoth C, Schultz N, et al. Integrated genomic characterization of endometrial carcinoma. Nature 2013;497:67–73.
6. Cancer Genome Atlas Research Network, Weinstein JN, Collisson EA, et al. The Cancer Genome Atlas Pan-Cancer analysis project. Nat Genet 2013;45:1113–20.
7. Davis CF, Ricketts CJ, Wang M, et al. The somatic genomic landscape of chromophobe renal cell carcinoma. Cancer Cell 2014;26:319–30.
8. Hoadley KA, Yau C, Wolf DM, et al. Multiplatform analysis of 12 cancer types reveals molecular classification within and across tissues of origin. Cell 2014;158:929–44.
9. Pantanowitz L, Tuthill JM, Balis UGJ. Pathology Informatics: Theory and Practice. Canada: ASCP Press; 2012.
10. Hogeweg P. The roots of bioinformatics in theoretical biology. PLoS Comput Biol 2011;7:e1002021.
11. Yu U, Lee SH, Kim YJ, et al. Bioinformatics in the post-genome era. J Biochem Mol Biol 2004;37:75–82.
12. Gargis AS, Kalman L, Berry MW, et al. Assuring the quality of next-generation sequencing in clinical laboratory practice. Nat Biotechnol 2012;30:1033–6.
13. Rehm HL, Bale SJ, Bayrak-Toydemir P, et al. ACMG clinical laboratory standards for next-generation sequencing. Genet Med 2013;15:733–47.
14. Mattocks CJ, Morris MA, Matthijs G, et al. A standardized framework for the validation and verification of clinical molecular genetic tests. Eur J Hum Genet 2010;18:1276–88.
15. Praxton A. CAP leads way with next-gen checklist. CAP Today 2012.
16. Sanger F, Nicklen S, Coulson AR. DNA sequencing with chain-terminating inhibitors. Proc Natl Acad Sci U S A 1977;74:5463–7.
17. Mullis KB, Faloona FA. Specific synthesis of DNA in vitro via a polymerase-catalyzed chain reaction. Methods Enzymol 1987;155:335–50.
18. Mardis ER. Next-generation sequencing platforms. Annu Rev Anal Chem (Palo Alto Calif) 2013;6:287–303.
19. Xuan J, Yu Y, Qing T, et al. Next-generation sequencing in the clinic: promises and challenges. Cancer Lett 2013;340:284–95.
20. Cottrell CE, Al-Kateb H, Bredemeyer AJ, et al. Validation of a next-generation sequencing assay for clinical molecular oncology. J Mol Diagn 2014;16:89–105.

21. Nikiforov YE, Carty SE, Chiosea SI, et al. Highly accurate diagnosis of cancer in thyroid nodules with follicular neoplasm/suspicious for a follicular neoplasm cytology by ThyroSeq v2 next-generation sequencing assay. Cancer 2014; 120(23):3627–34.

22. Pritchard CC, Salipante SJ, Koehler K, et al. Validation and implementation of targeted capture and sequencing for the detection of actionable mutation, copy number variation, and gene rearrangement in clinical cancer specimens. J Mol Diagn 2014;16:56–67.

23. Singh RR, Patel KP, Routbort MJ, et al. Clinical validation of a next-generation sequencing screen for mutational hotspots in 46 cancer-related genes. J Mol Diagn 2013;15:607–22.

24. Pabinger S, Dander A, Fischer M, et al. A survey of tools for variant analysis of next-generation genome sequencing data. Brief Bioinform 2014;15:256–78.

25. Ward JS, Barker A. Undefined by data: a survey of big data definitions. ArXiv e-prints; 2013. Available at: http://arxiv.org/abs/1309.5821. Accessed October 9, 2014.

26. Schneeweiss S. Learning from big health care data. N Engl J Med 2014;370: 2161–3.

27. Miriovsky BJ, Shulman LN, Abernethy AP. Importance of health information technology, electronic health records, and continuously aggregating data to comparative effectiveness research and learning health care. J Clin Oncol 2012;30: 4243–8.

28. Merelli I, Perez-Sanchez H, Gesing S, et al. Managing, analysing, and integrating big data in medical bioinformatics: open problems and future perspectives. Biomed Res Int 2014;2014:134023.

29. Grossman RL, White KP. A vision for a biomedical cloud. J Intern Med 2012;271: 122–30.

30. Heath AP, Greenway M, Powell R, et al. Bionimbus: a cloud for managing, analyzing and sharing large genomics datasets. J Am Med Inform Assoc 2014; 21(6):969–75.

31. Stein LD. The case for cloud computing in genome informatics. Genome Biol 2010;11:207.

32. Dove ES, Joly Y, Tasse AM, et al. Genomic cloud computing: legal and ethical points to consider. Eur J Hum Genet 2014. [Epub ahead of print].

33. U.S. Department of Health and Human Services: Health Information Privacy Rule. Available at: http://www.hhs.gov/ocr/privacy/hipaa/administrative/privacyrule/. Accessed October 9, 2014.

34. Modifications to the HIPAA Privacy, Security, Enforcement, and Breach Notification rules under the Health Information Technology for Economic and Clinical Health Act and the Genetic Information Nondiscrimination Act; other modifications to the HIPAA rules. Fed Regist 2013;78:5565–702.

Pathology Gross Photography
The Beginning of Digital Pathology

B. Alan Rampy, DO, PhD[a], Eric F. Glassy, MD[b],*

KEYWORDS

- Gross photography • Digital pathology • Electronic medical record
- Diagnostic report • Anatomic pathology

OVERVIEW: SETTING THE STAGE

Today, digital pathology equates to whole-slide imaging (WSI). But before high-priced scanners and computer-assisted diagnoses, there were static images of microscopic slides and gross surgical pathology specimens. This is where digital pathology started. Photomicrography has given way to WSI but capturing and documenting gross surgical pathology specimens is just as important and, the authors argue, a key component of the pathology report and the electronic medical record.

AP is a visual discipline and photographic documentation of clinical specimens is an essential element of the effective practice of pathology. Because photography is not a fundamental subject of medical training, pathology residents most often have little experience with photography as it applies to the AP setting. Moreover, whereas there seems to be broad consensus that basic digital gross pathology competency should be considered a requisite component of pathology education[1] and is accordingly included in the list of training objectives and residency handbooks of most major residency programs, available learning resources are scant. Of the publications with regard to gross pathology photography, most address the logistics of image acquisition, transfer, and storage or the relative benefits of select hardware/software advances.[2–6] As such, only a few articles serve as essential guides to understanding the importance of hands-on strategies and techniques for quality gross photography.[7–10] The aim of this article is to describe informally, through a variety of examples, many of the important concepts that underlie quality gross pathology photography.

This article originally appeared in Surgical Pathology Clinics, Volume 8, Issue 2, June 2015.
Disclosures: Dr B.A. Rampy: Medical Advisory Board: Xifin, Inc; Dr E.F. Glassy: Consultant: Leica Biosystems, PersonalizeDx; Advisory Board: Definiens; and Minority cOwnership: Pathology, Inc (reference laboratory).
[a] Department of Pathology, University of Texas Medical Branch, 301 University Boulevard, Mail Route 0747, Galveston, TX 77555-0747, USA; [b] Affiliated Pathologists Medical Group, 19951 Mariner Avenue #155, Torrance, CA 90503, USA
* Corresponding author.
E-mail address: efglassymd@affiliatedpath.com

GROSS PHOTOS IN PRACTICE

Quality gross specimen photographs are a fundamental element of AP practice. Such images not only are part of patient medical records but also are often reviewed at conferences, used as educational material, and integrated into professional publications. The value of thoughtful, complete, and first-rate image support cannot be overstated. Photos obtained by a prosector assigned to a particular case are often the only permanent record of specimen features and associated anatomic landmarks, prior to histopathologic sampling. As pathology practices merge and cases are handed off to others at sign-out, the need for visual documentation of complicated surgical specimens becomes even more critical. A related benefit of gross photography may be realized at microscopic examination, whereupon photographic review may be used to map sites of histologic sections. In addition to multidisciplinary review of digital pathology WSI at tumor board conferences in select institutions, it is expected that relevant gross pathology photographs will be available for assessment as well. Pathology practice is also part of the broad realm of patient-centered care, health information sharing, and electronic medical records, and, with ever increasing frequency, pathology gross photography is considered for integration into AP laboratory information systems, electronic medical records, and pathology diagnostic reports.[11] This guide for gross pathology imaging would not be complete without mention of the critical importance of associated specimen/patient information. Just as many experienced pathologists have desk drawers full of 35-mm photographic slides identified only by a specimen accession number, quality digital gross images are only of value if they are stored and archived along with appropriate metadata. Given these considerations, along with thoughtful attention to optimized patient care, clinical concerns, and associated educational opportunities, any pathology laboratory may establish a standard of excellence for gross specimen photography.

THE DECISION TO SHOOT

Not every gross specimen needs to be photographed. A good guideline to determine whether a specimen should be photographed is simple—all grossly evident pathology should be documented. Following this basic rule, if and when a clinical request for gross presentation of a particular specimen is received, the relevant pathology images may be reliably and readily provided. But that is not quite all. The photos should be taken to best show any and all associated disease processes, and the photos should be aimed to address all relevant clinical questions and concerns. Additionally, all grossly absent yet expected pathologic features should be documented in the photo records. Moreover, when the issue may be of particular clinical importance, photos should document the appearance of the specimen as it was received in pathology, before any further manipulations have taken place. For clarity, it is generally a good idea to orient a series of photographs of the same specimen in the same way. Consider photographing specimens that have sutures or other surgical markings in a manner that corresponds to the description, such as "short suture superior" at the top of the photo. Each set of images should tell a story, so that the final composite leads to a conclusion.

Because gross-only specimens, by definition, have no tissue submitted for histology, and hence no associated histologic diagnosis, complete quality photo documentation is imperative. This means that gross-only specimens should be photographed from all perspectives and all clinically relevant details should be included. Explanted medical devices, such as breast implants, intrauterine devices, and catheters, are a special subset of gross-only specimens and should be treated as such. These devices should be examined thoroughly and additional photos should document all identifying features like brand name and serial number as well as any probable sites of defect. As with medical devices, any specimens that, based on clinical history, likely will have medicolegal action should be documented thoroughly. They should be photographed from all perspectives, with attention to any clinically relevant details. If the specimen is patient derived and associated with trauma, thoroughly document associated pathologic changes, which may include such features as hemorrhage, lacerations, and so forth as well as any foreign material present (bullets, grass, gravel, and the like). Last but certainly not least, thoroughly document all unusual or rare specimens with photos from all perspectives, and be certain to include characteristic features of the pathology involved, because these shots may serve as valuable material for students, pathologists in training, and clinicians.

Although a vermiform appendix is most often considered a simple and routine surgical specimen, photos should document the associated grossly evident pathology. As shown in **Fig. 1**, with markedly congested vessels along the serosa and a tan to olive-green suppurative exudate, this gross image readily supports the diagnosis of acute gangrenous appendicitis and periappendicitis. **Fig. 2** is a gross image of another vermiform appendix submitted to surgical pathology with the clinical diagnosis of acute appendicitis. This specimen should likewise be well documented with photographs. There is no evident pathology present. Yet, because the appendix was submitted with clinical diagnosis of acute appendicitis, this discrepancy must be clearly demonstrated in the associated gross photos. A segment of rib submitted as a gross-only specimen is presented in **Fig. 3**. This segment of rib was received in surgical pathology as a routine, incidental element of a radical nephrectomy. As such, the rib is considered a gross-only specimen. Whereas there is no grossly evident pathology, other than that associated with the surgical manipulation, it should be photographed from both anterior and posterior perspectives to document the essentially normal appearance. An explanted breast implant specimen is a special type of gross-only specimen, because it is considered a medical device (**Fig. 4**). Hence, it should be handled with the routine protocol for such items—photographed from all perspectives to fully document the appearance of the device and with additional images to record any identifiers, such as the "225" text seen on one aspect. The

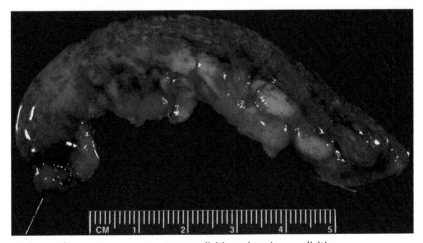

Fig. 1. Appendix: acute gangrenous appendicitis and periappendicitis.

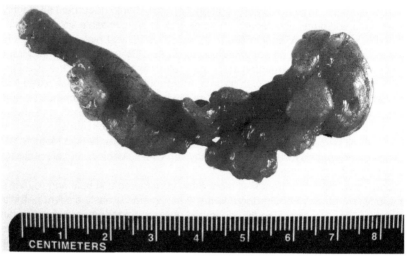

Fig. 2. Appendix: no pathologic change.

pathology evident in the specimen of **Fig. 5** is exclusively that associated with trauma and should be thoroughly documented, because such images support the clinical history of traumatic amputation—a history that potentially raises the probability of subsequent medicolegal concerns. The specimen presented in **Fig. 6** is a remarkable example of a solitary fibrous tumor, as seen in a transverse section of lung. Appearance during gross handling may suggest that a specimen warrants particularly comprehensive gross photography. This most often occurs when a specimen appears, through gross examination, to be unusual or rare or, in contrast, is a classic example of a common pathologic finding.

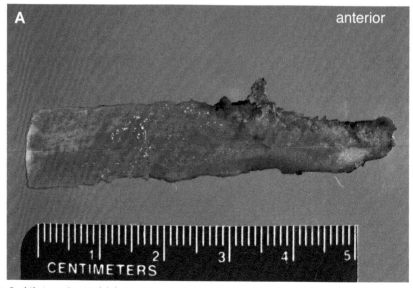

Fig. 3. (*A*) Anterior and (*B*) posterior aspects of gross-only rib specimen.

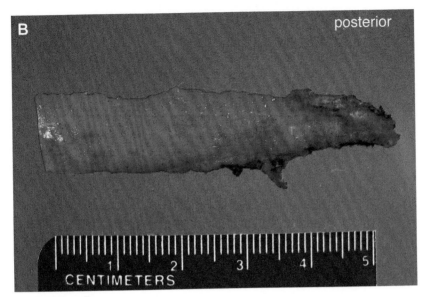

Fig. 3. (*continued*)

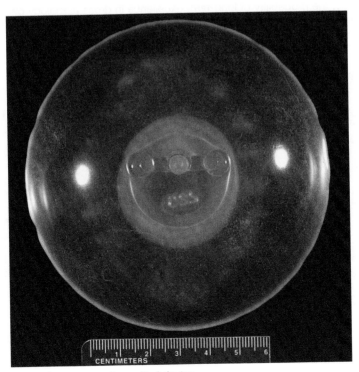

Fig. 4. Breast implant gross-only medical device.

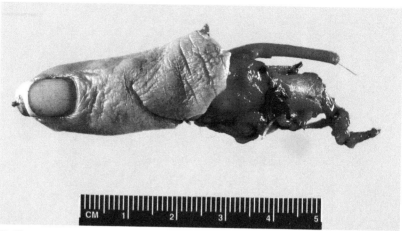

Fig. 5. Finger status post traumatic amputation.

THE SETUP

If at all possible, a small room should be dedicated to the gross pathology photography setup. Specific photographic equipment, accessories, and configuration will no doubt be driven by space and budgetary constraints, but a few guidelines are suggested. Almost without exception, the prosectors or personnel expected to obtain the appropriate, high-quality gross photographs are busy with other clinical demands. Accordingly, the probability of long-term excellence in gross pathology photography is most strongly predicted by the ease of use and time required for obtaining the desired images.

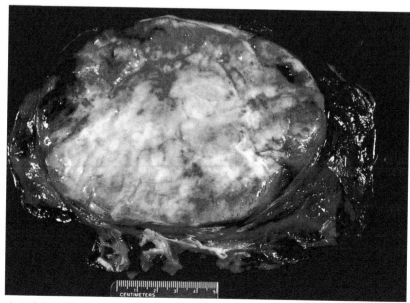

Fig. 6. Left lung: solitary fibrous tumor (transverse section).

Use of a small, dedicated room for gross photography activities allows for the control of one of the most common complications observed with routine gross photography (**Fig. 7**). A basic, user-friendly gross pathology photography stand may be configured with only a few pieces of routine photographic equipment. A sturdy, broad-based table frame may serve as an excellent foundation for a column copy stand of at least 40 inches with an adjustable camera arm and table-mounted copy stand lights with diffusion. Secured atop the table, a specimen stage may be fashioned from a strong, glass-topped, shallow box case (**Fig. 8**). With this case positioned at a comfortable height, background colors may be easily interchanged by placement of colored mat boards inside the open front face of the box case.

To minimize vibration and image blur, as well as to minimize direct handling of the camera during gross photography, use a shutter release cable or a wireless remote shutter control. Moreover, as a means of real-time quality control, always review the just-captured images of gross specimens, so that if necessary, adjustments may be made and new photos obtained while the material is readily available. To achieve this end, a remote monitor for the camera greatly simplifies the tasks of image review

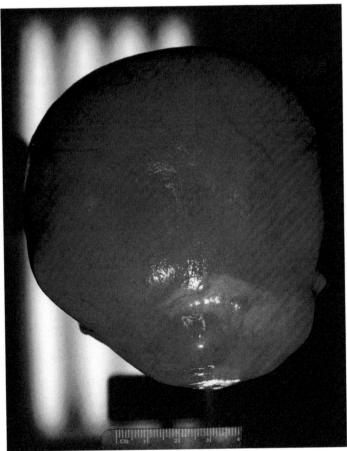

Fig. 7. Reflection of overhead fluorescent lights is a distraction in this external image of a markedly enlarged ovary.

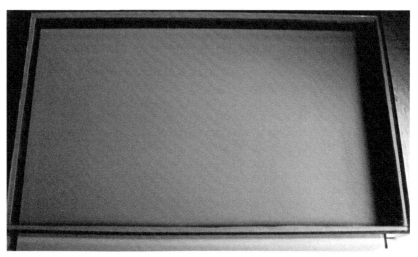

Fig. 8. Glassed-topped box with open front slot for easy placement of background mat boards.

for framing, focus, and exposure compared with appraisal using the small camera screen.

In the setting of AP photography, it is imperative to regularly clean the camera lens with lens cleaning solution and a cleaning cloth. This section through a pneumonectomy specimen (**Fig. 9**) documents a good example of squamous cell carcinoma, except that the area just left of center is visually soft and somewhat blurred due to a smudge on the camera lens. Likewise, prepare any specimen to be photographed. Surfaces should be wiped clean of blood, and other material, such as tubes or bandages, should be removed. In **Fig. 10**, the photo stand glass, often called the

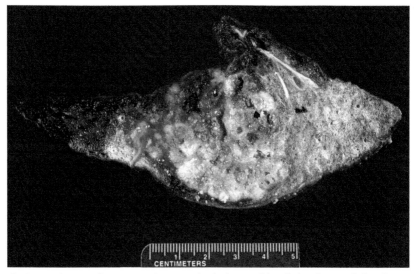

Fig. 9. A smudge on the camera lens results in image blur (left of center) for this cross-section of pneumonectomy specimen.

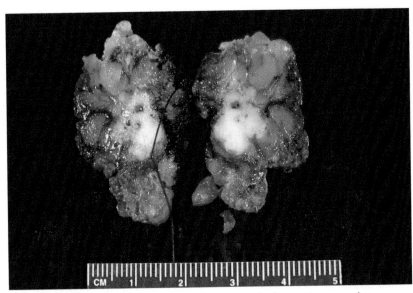

Fig. 10. The specimen stage is smeared in this image of a lumpectomy specimen.

specimen stage, is smeared such that it distracts from this photo of a lumpectomy specimen, which exhibits a tan irregular mass subsequently diagnosed as ductal carcinoma in situ. Similarly, the quality presentation of this example of a cross-section through a neurofibroma (**Fig. 11**) is greatly diminished by the presence of a surgical suture draped across the cut surface. Whereas routine specimen preparation is an essential step for general photo quality, if clinically relevant, additional photo documentation may be essential to record the state of a specimen as it was received in

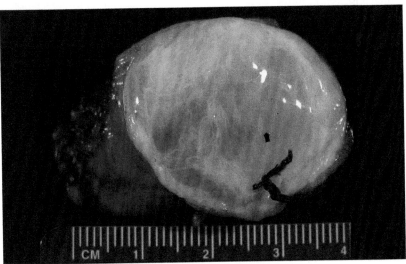

Fig. 11. Lack of specimen preparation results with a surgical suture across the surface of this cross-section of a neurofibroma.

pathology. This photo of a segment of umbilical cord with a true knot (**Fig. 12**) demonstrates the state of the specimen "as is" or as it was received in pathology and illustrates a clinically relevant feature. Regardless of specimen type, clinical concerns, or questions, always aim to capture as much detail as possible, and, accordingly, take the time and effort to position a specimen and the camera such that the entire specimen (or particular regions of interest) fills most of the available frame. Failure to attend to this exceedingly important facet of photographic documentation often results in images of little or no value to patients or any of the associated stakeholders (**Fig. 13**). A collection of poor photo techniques is shown in **Fig. 14**.

THE TOOLS

Choose an appropriate background to highlight specimen details. Black is a reasonable choice for many specimens (**Fig. 15**) and moreover may mask small smudges or drops of fluid on the specimen stage. Black, however, is typically a poor choice for dark brown or dark red specimens, like liver and spleen or any specimens that exhibit blood covered surfaces. In general, red, yellow, and brown are most often poor background selections for routine specimens, whereas, in contrast, light blue (**Fig. 16**) and light green (**Fig. 17**) are colors that enhance overall image presentations. But red may be a good choice for slices of fixed brain sections (see **Fig. 18**). If using just a cloth background, consider wetting the cloth first to enhance the contrast and reduce the texture of the cloth. Given these recommendations, in pathology practice, background selections are often driven by personal preference, resources, or particular camera characteristics.

It is generally accepted that most pathology gross photos should include a scale and label, identified with the specimen accession number. In the frame of the image, the scale should be placed inferior to yet near the specimen. Not only does such placement contribute to an ease of interpretation for specimen gross morphology but also this arrangement simplifies the task of photo editing (removing accession number or other identifiers), if the image is to be shared in presentation or publication. The scale should not be placed on the specimen or obstruct the view of any part of the specimen (**Fig. 18**). To further assist the viewer of gross pathology photos, employ the following sensible guidelines. If a specimen is large, use an entire standard 15-cm scale for reference (**Fig. 19**). Whereas, if a specimen is small, just a few centimeters

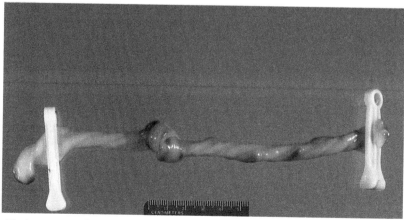

Fig. 12. A segment of umbilical cord is photographed as is.

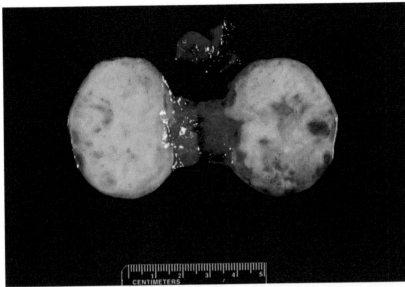

Fig. 13. A poorly framed image of a mildly enlarged ovary results from the camera at too great distance from the specimen and lacks morphologic detail.

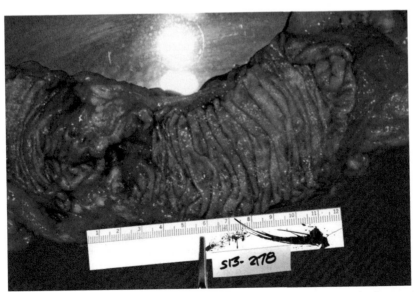

Fig. 14. This gross photo suffers from multiple composition errors. The background is marred by reflected lighting, the label and ruler are askew, the ruler has a prominent logo and is smeared with blood, and the alligator clip from the third hand (see **Fig. 20**) is also visible, the scale overlies and obscures part of the specimen. The specimen label is hand-written and legible, but a printed label is preferable.

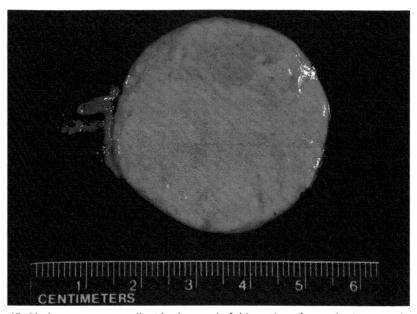

Fig. 15. Black serves as an excellent background of this section of an amber/orange adrenal cortical adenoma.

or less, cut the scale to a length slightly longer than the specimen (**Fig. 20**). This greatly aids with visually approximating specimen-related dimensions. And, as another service to the viewer, be sure to include the zero point and the unit of measure designation, usually centimeters, in the segments of the scale cut to size. As nearly as can be approximated, place the scale with the associated label in the plane of focus for the specimen. This may be readily accomplished with the use of a "third hand" (**Fig. 21**) to hold the scale with label at the appropriate plane of focus while remaining out of the image frame. A plastic pointer or metal probe may also be attached to indicate a particular area of interest (discussed later). Such a device was used during the capture of many of the images for this article. Another option is to use a wooden holder, made from a slide box, that allows the height of a ruler and label attached to a glass slide to be readily adjusted (**Fig. 22**). Once a gross photo appropriately identifies a specimen with a scale and label, any additional close-up photos or macrophotos of a portion of the same field of view need not be accompanied by the label and scale. As for rulers, it is important not to include any logos or marketing text that distract from the effective presentation of the specimen. Rolls of disposable rulers that may be attached to a glass slide are also available.

The number and wide variety of digital cameras available for gross imaging are remarkably extensive and a detailed discussion is not possible in this article. Some of these cameras capture images that may be readily and directly imported into an AP laboratory information system, whereas others require wireless or manual transfer from a memory card. An LED lighting system often yields superior images compared with flash photography. Even without a dedicated photo setup, the best camera is the one with ready access, which often may be a mobile smartphone. These multiuse devices often have the capacity to capture excellent macroimages, usually without a flash, derived through use of the built-in camera or by attaching high-quality lenses,

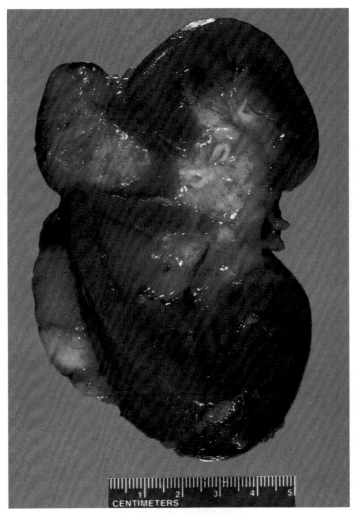

Fig. 16. Light blue serves as an excellent background for most specimen types and colors and provides a nice contrast to the dark red tissue of this section of kidney with a small tan/pink angiomyolipoma positioned near the upper left.

such as the Olloclip, to smartphones. Waterproof cases are also available for many cameras and smartphones, which may offer the benefit of keeping the phone clean.

THE CLUES

As specimens are handled and processed, attention must be directed to the associated clinical concerns and questions, such that important photos are obtained at various stages of sectioning. Often, intact organs reveal little of the pathologic changes that lie deep within the specimen. Always remember to photograph the appropriate cut surfaces, which reveal specimen structural architecture, and associated relations to any evident pathologic features. **Fig. 23**A reflects a perfectly adequate image of a markedly enlarged ovary. This grossly evident pathology should

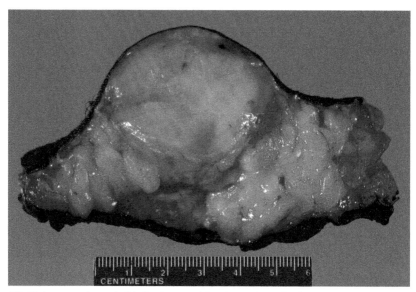

Fig. 17. Light green is a suitable background for the variety of colors seen in this section of a dermatofibrosarcoma protuberans, which exhibits a darkly pigmented skin surface, a light tan neoplasm, yellow adipose tissue, and specimen margin inks, including black along the deep margin and orange to the right.

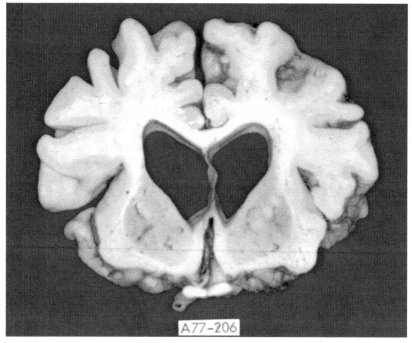

Fig. 18. Brain section showing hydrocephalus. Normally red is a poor background for gross surgical pathology specimens, but for brain slices, the red cloth background creates a pleasing contrast to the pale neural tissue. The cloth was first wetted down and smoothed out before laying the brain section on top.

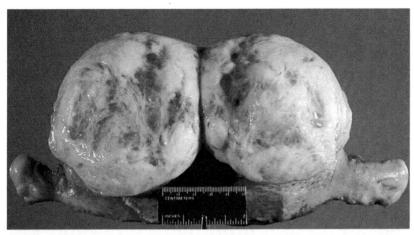

Fig. 19. A scale obscures the view of a portion of the uterine wall in this bivalved hysterectomy specimen with a large leiomyoma.

be photographed, yet little detail with regard to the associated specific pathologic process may be determined from this superficial photograph. A cross-section of the ovary (see **Fig. 23B**) does much to reveal diagnostic features of this neoplasm. The solid, yellow-tan whorled cut surface is characteristic of a fibrothecoma and thus should be included in the photographic history for this specimen. When shooting a sectioned specimen, if 2 or more slices exhibit essentially the same features, photograph 1 individually, so as to more closely frame the specimen and best demonstrate the gross pathology. Note again, in **Fig. 23B**, this lesion is homogeneous throughout; hence, photographing this one-half of the specimen is, in this instance, more effective than presenting both (essentially identical) cut surfaces side by side.

To draw attention to a focal region of interest, an appropriately positioned probe may be used to highlight the significant area while minimally obstructing the view of the overall specimen. Such an approach is used to great effect in **Fig. 24**, wherein a localization needle, submitted with a breast lumpectomy specimen, serves to direct attention to a small focus of ductal carcinoma in situ. Moreover, such an approach

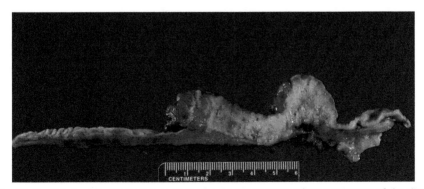

Fig. 20. For this longitudinal cross-section of a deeply invasive adenocarcinoma of the distal esophagus, the segment of scale is not even as long as the lesion of interest and certainly too short to readily estimate overall gross dimensions.

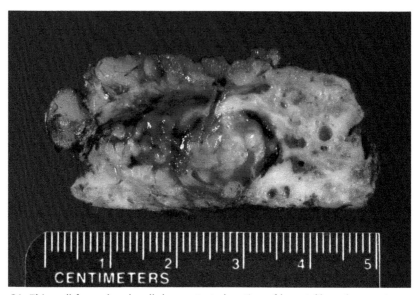

Fig. 21. This well-framed and well-demonstrated section of breast fibroadenoma is accompanied by a scale segment that affords easy translation to the overall specimen and internal elements.

is particularly useful for demonstrating narrow channels through specimens, such as sinus tracts, perforations, and so forth (**Fig. 25**). Another method to best emphasize the gross architecture of delicate specimens is to photograph them floating in saline. The liquid helps support delicate tissue architecture, as is often present with small papillary and cystic structures. With this approach, the best images are obtained with the specimen transilluminated from below or from the sides (**Fig. 26**). In certain circumstances the best gross photo may not be derived from a customary camera mounted on a photo stand. A seldom-used yet often effective alternative technique for gross photography is derived through the use of a digital flatbed scanner. With limited specimen preparation and scanner configuration to optimize lighting and background,[12,13] specimens with intricate 3-D structure and depth (field of view) of up to a 0.5 cm or more may yield high-quality detailed images (**Fig. 27**). A final strategy is sometimes useful in the unfortunate incidence that an important photograph of a specimen was not obtained in the fresh state. To somewhat restore or refresh the original colors of a specimen that has been formalin fixed, place it from 1 to a few hours in 100% ethanol. Results vary greatly depending on the tissue type and the duration of prior fixation, but for obtaining a gross image for special circumstances, the protocol is usually worth a try (**Fig. 28**).

THE POINT

Contemporary AP practice is abuzz with the many exciting new opportunities associated with WSI, quantitative image analysis, telepathology, and other digital pathology techniques. Nonetheless, the well-established practice of photographing AP specimens, whether from surgical pathology or autopsy, continues to be of invaluable benefit to patients, clinicians, pathologists, and students. As such, this time-honored convention—the true beginning of digital pathology—will continue to afford

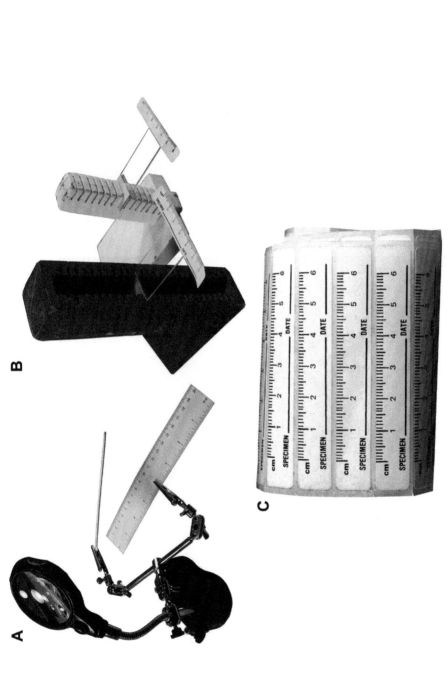

Fig. 22. The image on the top left (A) shows a third hand, which consists of movable arms at the end of which are alligator clips. The clips can hold a scale, a probe, or other item at an appropriate position. At the top right (B) are 2 wooden slide holders. The glass slide can be positioned within the grooves to put the ruler and label at the correct focal point. Also, the glass slide is not visible if it is in the frame of the photograph. On the bottom (C) is a roll of paper rulers.

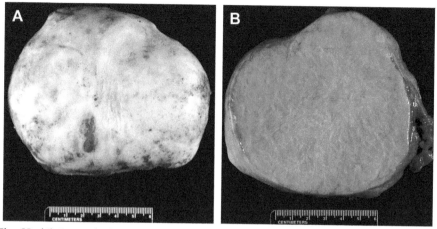

Fig. 23. (*A*) External photograph of an enlarged ovary reveals only superficial features, whereas (*B*) this cross-section of the ovary reveals the characteristic gross features of a fibrothecoma.

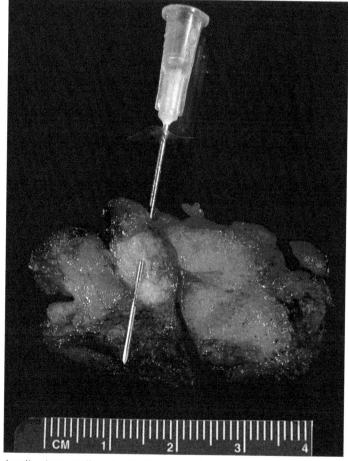

Fig. 24. A localization needle submitted with this lumpectomy is included to direct attention to a small focus of ductal carcinoma in situ.

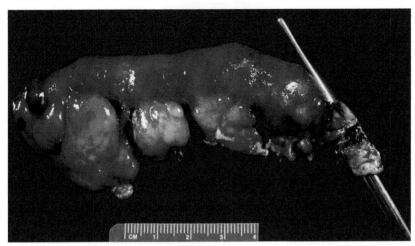

Fig. 25. A fundamental element of this photo of a vermiform appendix with gangrenous appendicitis is the placement of a probe that localizes an associated site of perforation.

unique advantages alongside the newer and developing imaging solutions. The widespread integration of digital photography into routine pathology workflow has almost eliminated turnaround time for availability of gross pathology images and has also greatly flattened the learning curve required for users to obtain excellent photos. With a limited set of hardware resources and effort, and following a few basic guidelines as set forth in this article, any AP practice may expect a standard of excellence in gross pathology photography.

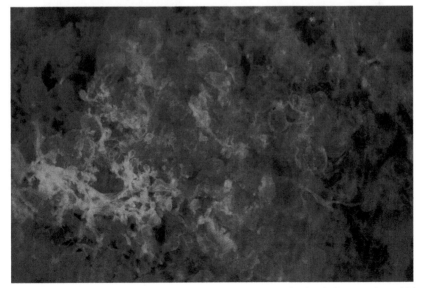

Fig. 26. The specimen for this striking photo is a complete hydatidaform mole, which is floated in saline to better demonstrate the innumerable, delicate, cystic grapelike villi, which are a characteristic feature.

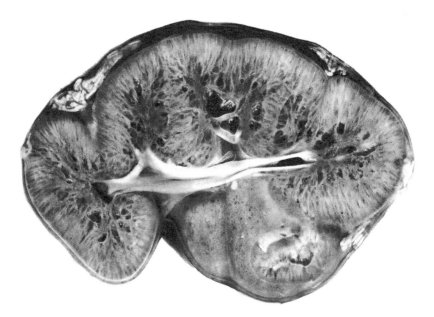

Fig. 27. Remarkable morphologic detail is exhibited in this image acquired with a commercial flatbed scanner of a longitudinal hemisection of formalin-fixed kidney with infantile polycystic kidney disease.

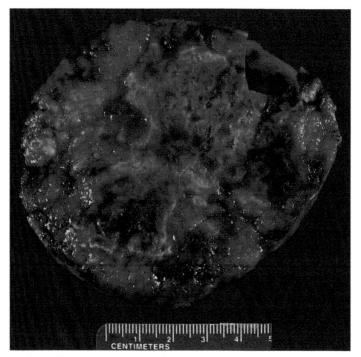

Fig. 28. This photo illustrates the result of an attempt to simulate the fresh appearance of this slice from a previously formalin-fixed ovarian mass, a Sertoli-Leydig cell tumor. After several hours in 100% ethanol, the tan-brown fixed section refreshed with a more tanpink to red appearance, somewhat similar to the original fresh appearance. Because this was a previously sectioned specimen, note the territory of absent tissue in the upper right.

REFERENCES

1. Wright JR, Spitalnik SL. Digital Pathology Workshop Proceedings from the Association of Pathology Chairs 2002 Annual Meeting. Available at: http://www.apcprods.org/Meetings/2002/index.cfm. Accessed March 5, 2015.
2. Campbell GA. Imaging, image analysis and computer-assisted quantitation: applications for electronic imaging in pathology. In: Cowen D, editor. Informatics for the clinical laboratory: a practical guide for the pathologist. New York: Springer; 2002. p. 251–67.
3. Hamza SH, Reddy VV. Digital image acquisition using a consumer-type digital camera in the anatomic pathology setting. Adv Anat Pathol 2004;11(2):94–100.
4. Park RW, Eom JH, Byun HY, et al. Automation of gross photography using a remote-controlled digital camera system. Arch Pathol Lab Med 2003;127:726–31.
5. Leong FJ, Leong AS. Digital photography in anatomic pathology. J Postgrad Med 2004;50(1):62–9.
6. Riley RS, Ben-Ezra JM, Massy E, et al. Digital photography: a primer for pathologists. J Clin Lab Anal 2004;18:91–128.
7. Finkbeiner WE, Ursell PC, Davis RL. Autopsy photography and radiology. In: Finkbeiner WE, Ursell PC, Davis RL, editors. Autopsy pathology: a manual and atlas. 2nd edition. Philadelphia: Saunders Elsevier; 2009. p. 81–6.
8. Lester SC. Microscopy and photography. In: Lester SC, editor. Manual of surgical pathology. 3rd edition. Philadelphia: Saunders Elsevier; 2010. p. 215–6.
9. Rosai J. Gross techniques in surgical pathology. In: Rosai J, Ackerman L, editors. Rosai and Ackerman's surgical pathology. 10th edition. Edinburgh (United Kingdom): Mosby Elseveir; 2011. p. 31.
10. Barker N. Photography. In: Westra WH, Hruban RH, Phelps TH, et al, editors. Surgical pathology dissection: an illustrated guide. 2nd edition. New York: Springer; 2003. p. 26–32.
11. Amin M, Sharma G, Parwani AV, et al. Integration of digital gross pathology images for enterprise-side access. J Pathol Inform 2012;3:10.
12. Mai KT, Stinson WA, Burns BF, et al. Creating Digital Images of Pathology Specimens by using a Flatbed scanner. Histopathology 2001;39:323–5.
13. Matthews TJ, Denney PA. Digital imaging of surgical specimens using a wet scanning technique. J Clin Pathol 2001;54:326–7.

Advanced Imaging Techniques for the Pathologist

Jeffrey L. Fine, MD

KEYWORDS

- Advanced imaging • Digital pathology • Optical coherence tomography • OCT
- Digital pathology • In vivo microscopy • Ex vivo microscopy

OVERVIEW

This article discusses a group of novel imaging techniques that are exciting because they may disrupt traditional pathology diagnosis. Such technologies permit direct tissue imaging without delays for histology preparation or for slide scanning, which may mean that turnaround time for pathology diagnosis could radically diminish even if a pathologist is off-site. In vivo imaging is also a possibility, which might blur or diminish traditional boundaries between pathology and other medical specialties. Finally, this might represent a fabulous opportunity to fundamentally re-evaluate current surgical pathology practice, with more emphasis placed on creating clinically valuable tests versus traditional all-inclusive histopathology examination. There are unprecedented pressures related to simultaneously increasing clinical expectations and decreasing access to resources. It is the author's opinion that traditional pathology diagnosis may not continue to be feasible for all applications; brightfield microscopy may not be rapid enough or inexpensive enough despite its current status as gold standard for most histopathology diagnosis. Furthermore, nonpathology specialties are vigorously developing new clinical applications based on advanced imaging; if pathologists wish to be involved in such diagnostic efforts then proactive involvement is essential. Rather than present an exhaustive list of the various advanced imaging modalities,[1] an in-depth presentation of OCT is chosen. The aim is to present a pathologist-friendly introduction, so that interested pathologists will be better able to participate in these advanced imaging efforts.

This article originally appeared in Surgical Pathology Clinics, Volume 8, Issue 2, June 2015.
Disclosure: No conflicts of interest to report.
Subdivision of Advanced Imaging and Image Analysis (Pathology Informatics) Department of Pathology, University of Pittsburgh School of Medicine, 200 Lothrop Street, Pittsburgh, PA 15213, USA
E-mail address: finejl@upmc.edu

OPTICAL COHERENCE TOMOGRAPHY

OCT was originally developed more than 20 years ago and found its first application in ophthalmology,[2] with additional early work with blood vessel and gastrointestinal imaging.[3,4] There are many variants of OCT but it is generally understand that these mean differences in speed, resolution, tissue depth, and image orientation. Specifics are less important than understanding the general idea of what OCT is and how it could be used in a particular situation. Briefly, a specimen is illuminated and the reflected light is used to create a 2-D image or a stack of 2-D images that are virtual slices of the tissue (**Fig. 1**). An OCT image shows differences in reflectivity; nearly transparent tissues (eg, fat) reflect little light and are contrasted with other shinier tissues (**Fig. 2**). OCT can be simplistically explained by comparison with 3 other imaging techniques that may be more familiar: ultrasound, phase-contrast microscopy, and CT. The ultrasound similarity is easily understood, and that is reflection; ultrasound derives images from reflected sound, whereas OCT is based on light (**Table 1**). Unlike sound, light travels too quickly for direct time-based imaging so OCT images use interferometry, which is also used in phase-contrast microscopy. Although phase contrast is different from reflectivity, the overall configuration of an imager or microscope with a reference light path and interference-based imaging is similar.[5] OCT also features a

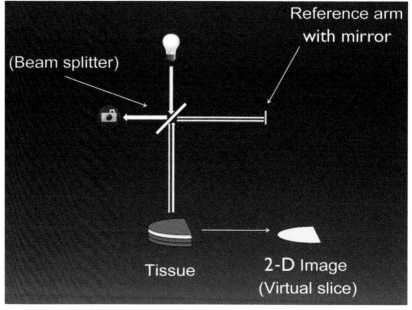

Fig. 1. OCT explained. Light is emitted from a source (*light bulb* and *yellow arrows*) and passes through a beam splitter. Some light travels along a reference arm and is reflected from a mirror back into the beam splitter (*more yellow arrows*). Some light travels into the tissue (*yellow arrow*), interacts with the tissue, and is then reflected back into the beam splitter (*white arrow*). Reflected light, both from reference arm and from tissue, combines in the beam splitter and undergoes interference. This interference pattern is imaged (*blue camera icon*) and is a 2-D image of the tissue due to the interaction of light with tissue. By varying the length of the reference arm, the imaged depth into the tissue can be varied. Depth is limited by the amount of reflected light; infrared light permits deeper imaging but offers less resolution than broad-spectrum visible light.

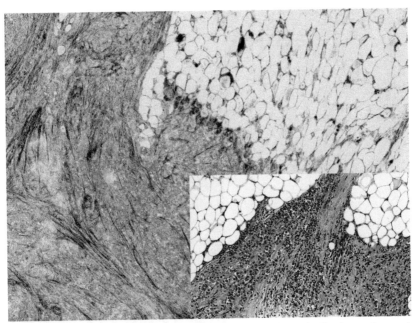

Fig. 2. Example OCT image (invasive lobular carcinoma of breast). The larger image is an OCT image of invasive lobular breast carcinoma with infiltration into fat. Fat is perhaps the most easily identified tissue due to the difference in reflectivity between cell membranes and cytoplasm of individual fat cells. The sharpness of the cell membranes visually conveys the high resolution of the image (approximately 1 μm per pixel in the original image). The inset H&E photomicrograph is derived from a WSI of the same tissue (approximately 0.5 μm per pixel, ×20 objective magnification). In the OCT image, individual tumor cell nuclei are visible as white spots in the gray background.

variable-length reference path for light, which means that variable tissue depths can be imaged into a tissue's surface. Imaging a series of images at different depths results in a stack of 2-D images, which can be viewed in sequence or can be reconstructed into a 3-D data set. This is like CT imaging, in that CT produces a stack of virtual slice radiographs that can be viewed in 2-D in multiple orientations or that can be used to create 3-D images (**Fig. 3**). OCT is also like CT in that it represents a data set that is too large to be viewed directly; viewable images represent subsets of the data. CT image viewers display portions of the data, using selective viewing recipes called windows (ie, bone window, soft tissue window, sinus window, brain

Table 1 Comparison of optical coherence tomography with other imaging modalities		
OCT	**Similarity**	**Difference**
Ultrasound	Reflection	OCT uses light, not sound
Phase-contrast microscopy	Interferometry	OCT shows reflectivity
CT	Virtual slices and 3-D data; images a subset of data	OCT has limited penetration into tissue depth

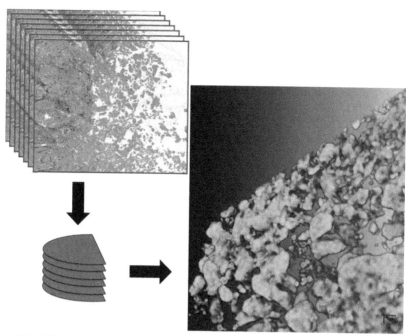

Fig. 3. 3-D OCT view of uterine papillary serous carcinoma. A series of OCT images were acquired from a hysterectomy specimen, from 1 field of view and at multiple tissue depths (*upper left corner*). These are stylistically shown as a stack of flat shapes (*lower left corner*). Using radiology (CT) software, a 3-D reconstruction view is created (*yellow/orange image to right*). Despite not being optimized for a pathology image, this clearly demonstrates the papillary architecture of the tumor.

window, and so forth). OCT images do not yet have such windows established but only because the images are so new to pathologists.

OCT image data sets can be large, although not as large as whole-slide images (WSIs). A single 2-D OCT slice of a frozen section block–sized piece of tissue, at 1-μm resolution, can be 20,000 by 10,000 pixels in size (more than 300 megabytes of raw data per slice). Such an image can be acquired in approximately 20 minutes with a current-generation OCT system without undue difficulty, but acquiring a stack of 150 to 200 such images would be infeasible due to time and computing constraints. A compromise is a series of few (eg, 3–5) levels, much like what is done with histopathology slides. Finally, manual review of such large image sets should optimally be augmented with software that helps detect clinically important areas, such as pathologists' computer-assisted diagnosis. One investigator team uses an OCT system to image large portions of the esophagus.[6] Such an image set is akin to totally submitting a specimen for H&E histology and then cutting many levels into each block—it would represent an enormous amount of image review if attempted manually. Therefore, the review should be targeted and augmented by computer assistance.

EXPERIENCE WITH OPTICAL COHERENCE TOMOGRAPHY

The author's earliest experience with OCT was the result of a collaboration with ophthalmologists.[7] Although this system only featured 20-μm resolution, it did not require contact with the specimen and, therefore, theoretically could be mounted vertically in a specimen grossing type of application, just as a conventional camera is deployed. Although not as good as a histology section, such OCT resolution permits seeing lesions, such as ductal carcinoma in situ (DCIS) in breast tissue, and may, therefore, be suitable for intraoperative margins assessment (**Fig. 4**). Furthermore, such an image does not require a cryostat, microscope, or the skill needed to obtain good frozen section histology on breast tissue. Finally, miniaturization of this type of device could eventually permit in vivo imaging from within an operating room; this should be of interest to surgeons because many procedures are now performed in outpatient surgical centers that do not have intraoperative support by pathologists, either on-site or remotely.

Another type of OCT imaging worth discussing in more detail, due to its high tissue resolution, is full-field OCT.[8] This imaging system is unique in that it is a pathology system that produces 2-D images at a 1-μm resolution, using oil-immersion microscopy on a tissue-block sized tissue piece inside a specimen holder (**Fig. 5**). This resolution is theoretically adequate for much diagnostic work and these images can often closely resemble medium-magnification H&E images, especially in tissues that contain cysts or lumens (**Fig. 6**). Such close correlation between OCT and H&E, however, represent a potential pitfall, because some lesions likely are difficult to see reliably without training and without targeted computer assistance (eg, image analysis and radiology-like windows). One good example is an image of vulvar Paget disease; if looked for, then squamous nuclei and Paget nests can easily be seen in the OCT image (**Fig. 7**). If there is not yet a diagnosis, then it is not clear that a pathologist could confidently make the diagnosis from OCT alone. The Paget lesion is visible, however, which means there is a diagnostic pattern in the OCT image data; in the author's opinion, this means that the OCT image can be diagnostic, but it will require more work to make this a reliable process. Breast tissue is another area that has been challenging due to inadequate contrast out of the box and despite good tissue resolution. Even subtle tumor infiltrates can retrospectively be seen but more work is needed to

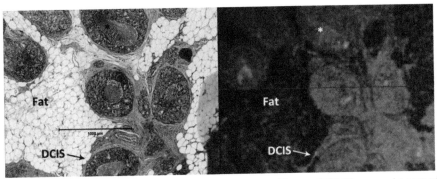

Fig. 4. Low-resolution OCT of DCIS. Side-by-side images of breast DCIS. These are images of the same area from a breast specimen: (*left*) H&E and (*right*) spectral domain OCT. The H&E image is from a WSI scanned at 0.5 μm per pixel (×20 objective magnification). The OCT image was acquired at approximately 20 μm per pixel using an ophthalmology device. Although higher-resolution OCT is possible, this device could be used to image breast tissue from a benchtop vantage point without special sample preparation (ie, just as with an conventional digital camera). Fat, DCIS and necrosis (*asterisk*) can clearly be identified in the OCT image; although perhaps not adequate for initial diagnosis, such an image might be useful for intraoperative assessment of margins.

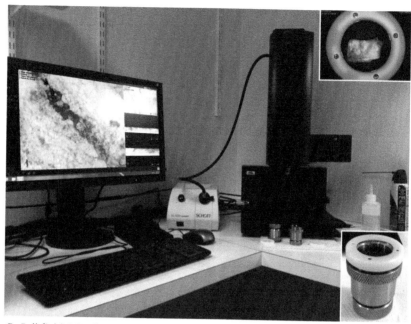

Fig. 5. Full-field OCT device. The main image is a photograph of a full-field OCT imaging system (Light-CT, LLTech, Paris, France). It use oil immersion microscopy with a ×10 objective and can image at 1 μm resolution in X, Y, and Z axes. It accommodates tissue block–sized tissue in a specimen holder (*inset, lower right corner*). Prior to OCT acquisition, a gross specimen scout image is also acquired (*inset, upper right corner*). This scout image permits driving about tissue in live mode prior to initiating a higher-quality permanent scan of the tissue.

make this a more reliable procedure for detection or identification of breast tumor cell infiltrates (**Fig. 8**).

Therefore, OCT images are not likely to be a direct replacement for traditional H&E histopathology for all tissues and for all clinical situations. In contrast to breast tissue, endometrium is extremely amenable to OCT imaging because there is already good contrast between glands, stroma, and myometrium without further image optimization. Although there will be a learning curve for interpretation of endometrial OCT images, it is already clear that pathologists can recognize structures just from their resemblance to known histopathology entities.[9] For example, in the author's own study, 3 pathologist subjects were able to distinguish benign versus malignant endometrium with a 10.44% discordance rate, despite having only 5 to 10 minutes of experience with an endometrial OCT image training set (**Figs. 9 and 10**).[10]

DISCUSSION

OCT is a powerful new imaging modality for pathologists. Although much early work took place in other medical specialties, OCT is microscopy and it produces images that are much more detailed than those typically interpreted by physicians in other specialties, such as radiology or gastroenterology. Pathologists are a natural choice for interpreting these images due to existing expertise not only with microscopy but also with test design and implementation. Although OCT images are unlikely to replace

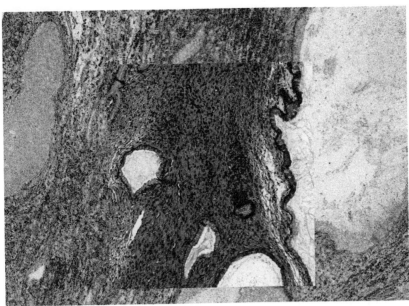

Fig. 6. OCT example (mucinous cystic ovary). This is an example of the high image quality that can be obtained with some specimens, such as this mucinous cystadenoma in an ovary (H&E image overlaid on top of OCT image). Glands versus stroma are easily discerned, and even the glandular cells' mucinous morphology is visible. Although H&E is more detailed, that image took much more time to create due to permanent section histology and WSI time requirements. The OCT image is a portion of a larger image that typically requires 10 to 20 minutes of acquisition time in this particular system (Light-CT, LLTech, Paris, France) (H&E image scanned at 0.5 μm objective resolution).

H&E histopathology, they are well suited to targeted clinical applications even with current-generation image quality (eg, intraoperative endometrial assessment). Therefore, development of advanced imaging applications may require a shift away from all-inclusive H&E diagnosis to narrower tests that address specific clinical questions. This is not without precedent; frozen section is a test that can quickly address clinical need without the expectation of definitive diagnosis (usually). Frozen section testing is generally bundled with a traditional H&E diagnosis, just as an OCT-based depth-of-invasion assessment in endometrial cancer is tied to subsequent histopathology review of the specimen. The real practice disruption likely will be from advanced imaging tests that are not bundled with a histology review. If pathologists wish to be involved in such testing, they should be actively engaged with clinical colleagues to identify unmet needs and other opportunities for rapid imaging diagnosis.

To this end, pathologist investigators need to work on building bridges between existing H&E histopathology and these new imaging techniques. Not only will such work permit new ex vivo applications but also it should also facilitate in vivo assessment. The previous example of vulvar OCT is a good example; the ability to make diagnoses in en face vulvar images could well translate into diagnosis on in vivo images from a gynecology office setting without a need for biopsy. Biopsy seems like a trivial procedure, but it does matter to patients. In vivo breast margin assessment is another good example and one that is being driven by breast surgeons.[11] Pathologists can be valued partners in these efforts, but it requires a proactive approach.

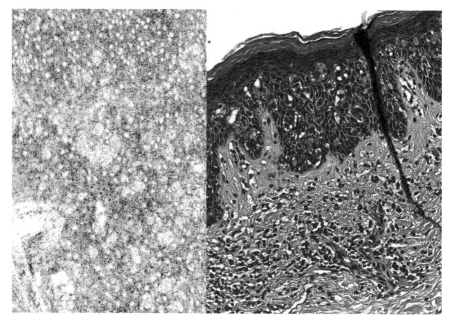

Fig. 7. Vulvar Paget disease. This is a side-by-side view of vulvar skin containing Paget disease: (*left*) OCT and (*right*) H&E. The OCT image was acquired en face from the skin surface, simulating a possible in vivo application. A population of smaller white round spots is clearly seen; these correlate with benign squamous cells. Larger irregular white blobs represent epidermal tumor nests of Paget cells. Although not well seen, in the lower left of the OCT image, a surface hair that is pressed between the vulvar skin and the imaging coverslip (shaped like an upside-down letter L) is clearly seen. The H&E image is a traditional section (eg, perpendicular to the surface) and shows the epidermis with small nests of Paget cells (H&E image scanned at 0.5 μm objective resolution).

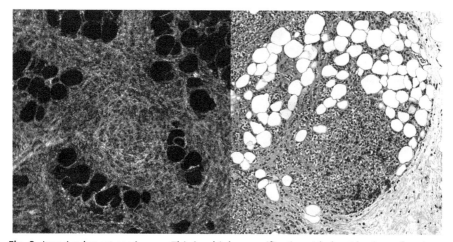

Fig. 8. Invasive breast carcinoma. This is a high-magnification side-by-side view of an invasive breast carcinoma: (*left*) OCT and (*right*) H&E. Tumor nuclei are clearly seen as small round dark shadows in the OCT image, and these correlate with the tumor nuclei in the H&E image. These are easily recognizable retrospectively, which means that pathologists and image analysis can be trained to find tumor in OCT images. This is an example of an OCT image, however, that is not ready-made for pathology diagnosis based on its superficial resemblance to the H&E image (H&E image scanned at 0.5 μm objective resolution).

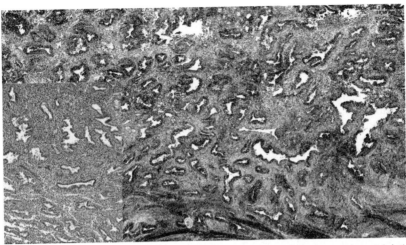

Fig. 9. Benign endometrium. This is a full-field OCT image of benign endometrial tissue (inset is an H&E image of the same tissue). The OCT and H&E images strongly resemble one another. Glands are readily seen because they contain lumens, but the glandular epithelium is also readily distinguished from endometrial stroma (H&E image scanned at 0.5 μm objective resolution).

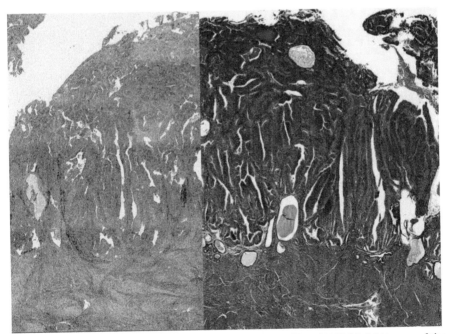

Fig. 10. Endometrial carcinoma. Low-magnification OCT (*left*) and H&E (*right*) images of the same endometrial tumor. The architecture of the glands is evident on OCT, as is the interface between endometrium and myometrium. Such images could be used for intraoperative assessment of endometrial tumor depth-of-invasion assessment and for confirmation of histology (H&E image scanned at 0.5 μm objective resolution).

Although current full-field OCT images may require 10 to 20 minutes of acquisition time, it is likely that refinements will lead to shorter imaging times just as has occurred with WSIs.[12] Therefore, timewise, OCT already compares favorably with frozen section, is much faster than routine histology, and does not require a separate slide-scanning step. OCT images may not require as much laboratory infrastructure to produce and could become an inexpensive method to project pathology expertise away from centralized laboratories.

Unfortunately, this short discussion cannot do justice to the ramifications of OCT and related direct tissue microscopy technologies, but these may be disruptive to the pathology status quo. In particular, in vivo diagnosis crosses into territory traditionally off-limits to laboratories. Such upending of the status quo may be a much-needed opportunity for pathologists to re-evaluate diagnostic practice fundamentally and even what it means to be a pathologist. This may already be happening as WSIs develop into clinical practice and as pathology groups seek to cope with an uncertain future.[13-15] Although H&E-based histopathology may remain a gold standard, it is possible that it will become too slow or too expensive in specific clinical situations. OCT and other advanced imaging may represent a way forward that permits responsive, excellent patient care despite decreased availability of resources.

REFERENCES

1. Chen Y, Liang CP, Liu Y, et al. Review of advanced imaging techniques. J Pathol Inform 2012;3:22.
2. Gabriele ML, Wollstein G, Ishikawa H, et al. Optical coherence tomography: history, current status, and laboratory work. Invest Ophthalmol Vis Sci 2011;52(5):2425–36.
3. Brezinski ME, Tearney GJ, Bouma BE, et al. Optical coherence tomography for optical biopsy: properties and demonstration of vascular pathology. Circulation 1996;93(6):1206–13.
4. Tearney GJ, Brezinski ME, Bouma BE, et al. In vivo endoscopic optical biopsy with optical coherence tomography. Science 1997;276(5321):2037–9.
5. Murphy DB, Oldfield R, Schwartz S, et al. Introduction to phase contrast microscopy. Nikon microscopy U (The source for microscopy education). Available at: http://www.microscopyu.com/articles/phasecontrast/phasemicroscopy.html. Accessed September 01, 2014.
6. Suter MJ, Vakoc BJ, Yachimski PS, et al. Comprehensive microscopy of the esophagus in human patients with optical frequency domain imaging. Gastrointest Endosc 2008;68(4):745–53.
7. Fine JL, Kagemann L, Wollstein G, et al. Direct scanning of pathology specimens using spectral domain optical coherence tomography: a pilot study. Ophthalmic Surg lasers Imaging 2010;41(Suppl):S58–64.
8. Jain M, Shukla N, Manzoor M, et al. Modified full-field optical coherence tomography: a novel tool for rapid histology of tissues. J Pathol Inform 2011;2:28.
9. Jain M, Narula N, Salamoon B, et al. Full-field optical coherence tomography for the analysis of fresh unstained human lobectomy specimens. J Pathol Inform 2013;4:26.
10. Cucoranu IC, Fine JL. Optical Coherence Tomography (OCT) for Intra-Operative Style Interpretation of Endometrium (USCAP Abstract, Informatics). Mod Pathol 2013;26:375–83.

11. Bydlon TM, Barry WT, Kennedy SA, et al. Advancing optical imaging for breast margin assessment: an analysis of excisional time, cautery, and patent blue dye on underlying sources of contrast. PLos One 2012;7(12):e51418.
12. Pantanowitz L, Valenstein PN, Evans AJ, et al. Review of the current state of whole slide imaging in pathology. J Pathol Inform 2011;2:36.
13. Cornish TC, Swapp RE, Kaplan KJ. Whole-slide imaging: routine pathologic diagnosis. Adv Anat Pathol 2012;19(3):152–9.
14. Kothari S, Phan JH, Stokes TH, et al. Pathology imaging informatics for quantitative analysis of whole-slide images. J Am Med Inform Assoc 2013;20(6): 1099–108.
15. Robboy SJ, Weintraub S, Horvath AE, et al. Pathologist workforce in the United States: I. Development of a predictive model to examine factors influencing supply. Arch Pathol Lab Med 2013;137(12):1723–32.

Overview of Telepathology

Navid Farahani, MD[a],*, Liron Pantanowitz, MD[b]

KEYWORDS

- Telepathology • Digital imaging • Robotic • Static • Teleconsultation
- Telemicroscopy • Virtual microscopy • Whole-slide imaging

OVERVIEW

Telepathology is the practice of pathology at a distance, transmitting macroscopic and/or microscopic images using telecommunication links for remote interpretations (telediagnosis), second opinions or consultations (teleconsultation), and/or for educational purposes.[1–4] The original material (eg, glass slide) is spatially separated from the remote consultant (telepathologist) who will interpret a representative image of the material. The digital or analog image is remotely viewed on a computer monitor or cell phone screen. Ubiquitous access to the Internet, or to other broadband telecommunications linkages, facilitates nearly global image sharing. As a result, telepathology has been used to aid a growing number of laboratories around the world to deliver pathology services by allowing them to easily connect with experts. Telepathology has even been used to enhance the efficiency of pathology services between hospitals less than a mile apart.[5,6] With increasing subspecialization in pathology, the use of telepathology to access subspecialists (eg, neuropathologists) has been extremely beneficial.[7–12] The practice of telepathology, however, is not only limited to diagnostic work but can be used in quality assurance (eg, rereview of cases), education, and research.[9,11]

The first recorded instance of "telepathology" occurred in the late 1960s, when a real-time "television microscopy" service was established between Massachusetts General Hospital (MGH) and Logan Airport Medical Station in Boston, Massachusetts.[13] Since then, there has been a proliferation of telepathology technology and services worldwide.[14,15] The number of "telepathology" citations indexed in MEDLINE has grown from the first citation listed in 1986 to 900 citations in 2015. The variety of telepathology systems developed and applications deployed continues to grow. To date, 12 distinct classes of telepathology systems have been described in the literature. These are listed in the Weinstein Telepathology System Classification, the primary modes of which are static imaging, dynamic imaging, and virtual slide

This article originally appeared in Surgical Pathology Clinics, Volume 8, Issue 2, June 2015.
[a] Department of Pathology and Laboratory Medicine, Cedars-Sinai Medical Center, Los Angeles, CA, USA; [b] Department of Pathology, University of Pittsburgh School of Medicine, Pittsburgh, PA, USA
* Corresponding author.
E-mail address: nfarahan@gmail.com

telepathology.[9] Despite the low equipment start-up costs, static image telepathology was slowly replaced by dynamic methods in an attempt to improve diagnostic accuracy.[16,17] With dynamic telepathology, the telepathologist is more actively involved in glass slide field selection, typically by using robotic, remote-controlled microscopy.[18–20] Virtual slide telepathology is the most recently developed mode of telepathology. This technology is also referred to as whole-slide imaging (WSI) telepathology. WSI systems produce giant, high-resolution, digital images of entire glass slides (ie, digital slides).[21] With disruptive WSI technology, innovative telepathology services have emerged.[12]

There are many potential uses of telepathology. Telepathology has been applied in anatomic pathology (eg, remote frozen section diagnosis, telecytology) and clinical pathology (eg, telehematology, telemicrobiology). Drawbacks to the widespread use of telepathology include cost, technology restrictions (eg, limited resolution, large image files), resistance from pathologists (eg, reluctance, skepticism, technophobia), lack of standards, and the potential threat of competition for pathology services. The development of standards for digital radiology imaging was critical to the success of teleradiology, and the same is likely to be true for telepathology. Standards for telepathology have begun to be developed, such as the recent guidelines set forth by the American Telemedicine Association.[22] The Canadian Association of Pathologists and Royal College of Pathologists also have published guidelines for telepathology.[23,24] Emerging legal and regulatory issues in telepathology also are being addressed, which will hopefully catalyze the practice of telepathology.[25]

TELEHEALTH

Telepathology falls under the broader category of telehealth. According to the Office for the Advancement of Telehealth, telehealth is defined as the use of electronic information and telecommunications technologies to support "long-distance" clinical health care, patient and professional health-related education, public health, and health administration. Telemedicine, another branch of telehealth, describes the remote transfer of clinical information via electronic communications.[3,26] Technologies used in telemedicine include the Internet, videoconferencing, store-and-forward imaging, streaming media, and wireless communications. Telemedicine can be further subdivided by specialty (eg, telepathology, teleradiology, teledermatology, telesurgery, telepsychiatry). The field of telemedicine is broad, because it also includes telerounding (eg, e-ICU "rounding"), telemonitoring (eg, home arrhythmia monitoring), televisits, telehome care, and telemanagement of patients.[27] Currently, most telemedicine programs consist of a central medical hub with several rural spokes, so as to improve access to services in underserved areas. Telehealth initiatives are growing due to lower costs of technology, federal funds supporting such programs, and advancements in technology.[28] Although the various branches of telehealth present unique opportunities for both patients and clinicians, they also possess distinct operational, ethical, and legal issues.[29] As the field grows, more standards and telepractice guidelines will be needed.[30]

HISTORICAL OVERVIEW

The history of telepathology has been long and eventful.[15,16,31] A list of several major milestones are provided in **Table 1**. The first telepathology event occurred in 1968, when black-and-white real-time television images of blood smears and urine specimens were sent from Logan Airport in Boston to the MGH for interpretation. In the 1990s, the value of telepathology for diagnosis was showcased by a landmark paper

Table 1
Historical telepathology milestones

Date	Historical Milestones
1968	Black-and-white photos of blood smears were sent via video from Logan Airport to the Massachusetts General Hospital in Boston
1980	Remote telepathology broadcasting demonstration on a commercial scale
1986	First video robotic telepathology system using satellite; introduction of the term "telepathology" into the English language; first telepathology patent application prepared for submission to the US Patent and Trademark Office with the patent granted in 1993
1989	Norway nationwide telepathology program established for frozen section services
1990	Published telepathology experience with more than 2200 VA hospital cases
1994	Hardware for a complete telepathology system becomes available
1995	AFIP static image consult service started
2000	WSI comes to market
2001	Dynamic telepathology used in the US Army Telemedicine Program
2005	US Army converts to WSI platform
2009	FDA panel meeting addresses the use of digital pathology for primary diagnosis
2011	Introduction of WSI dynamic-robotic/static imaging systems
2013	Telepathology guidelines developed by the Royal College of Pathologists
2014	Updated clinical guidelines for telepathology from ATA; published Canadian Association of Pathologists guidelines for establishing a telepathology service for anatomic pathology using WSI

Abbreviations: AFIP, Armed Forces Institute of Pathology; ATA, American Telepathology Association; FDA, Food and Drug Administration; VA, Department of Veterans Affairs; WSI, whole-slide imaging.

involving thousands of cases remotely interpreted at the Department of Veterans Affairs (VA) hospital in the United States.[17,32] Telepathology was used by VA hospitals for both anatomic pathology (eg, frozen sections) and clinical pathology services, without having a pathologist on-site at remote locations. The VA group involved in this study used an Apollo dynamic telepathology system, based on Weinstein and colleagues' robotic telepathology patents.[17,32] Their published data showed a high diagnostic concordance of robotic telepathology with light microscopy, and decreased turnaround time for surgical pathology cases at the remote site. By 2009, Dunn's group[17,32] had reported on their experience with over 11,000 telepathology cases. Pathologist-specific discordance rates using dynamic/robotic telepathology (0.12%–0.77%) were well below those noted using static image telepathology.[18,33,34]

Telepathology progress has typically been aligned with technologic advances. This evolution is nicely illustrated by the change of telepathology services that were offered by the US military. In 1993, the Armed Forces Institute of Pathology initiated a static imaging consult service in its pursuit of providing rapid expert consultation globally.[35] By 2001, dynamic telepathology was adopted by the US Department of Defense within the Army Telemedicine Program. In 2005, these systems were converted to a WSI platform. Since then, several companies have supplied competing products for digital imaging, providing users with an increasing range of scanning platforms and image viewers. Several commercial software solutions (eg, Corista, ePathAccess, Xifin) have started to build international networks, providing users and consulting groups with collaborative telepathology portals. These digital pathology networks provide virtual consultant consortiums with Web-enabled access to secure cloud services. With the growth of mobile health (mHealth) we are likely to witness greater use of telepathology using mobile devices (eg, tablets, cell phones, wearable glasses such as Google Glass).

TELEPATHOLOGY APPLICATIONS

Telepathology is currently most beneficial for providing pathology services to distant locations where the medical facilities lack on-site or easily accessible pathology services.[36] It is often logistically easier and cheaper to move an image around than it is to move a patient or pathologist. Telepathology can be used to expedite rapid consultation of remote cases where travel is not a viable option. It is also useful as a communication tool between general and sub-specialist pathologists.[5] Access to experts via telepathology, in which a teleconsultant remotely reviews digital images of challenging cases, has the potential to greatly improve patient care. In the appropriate setting, telepathology is therefore a cost-effective tool that ensures quick turnaround time, virtually eliminates expensive courier costs, improves resource utilization, permits load balancing, and creates added value.[37–39] **Table 2** highlights some of the advantages and disadvantages associated with telepathology applications.

Telepathology has been applied to all divisions of pathology, including surgical pathology, cytopathology, autopsy, and clinical pathology (especially hematopathology and microbiology).[40–43] Telepathology also has been used for sharing electron microscopic images,[44,45] and it has benefited veterinary medicine.[46] Telecytology, the practice of cytology at a distance, has been successful with both gynecologic specimens (eg, Pap tests) and nongynecological cases (eg, fine-needle aspirations).[47–54] Today, telecytology is mostly used for rapid on-site evaluation.[55] Diagnostic accuracy with telecytology is imperfect, and in early published studies ranged from 80% to 100%.[47,56] With improved technology (eg, robotic WSI scanners), diagnostic accuracy has

Table 2	
Clinical advantages and disadvantages associated with telepathology applications	
Advantages	**Disadvantages**
Primary Diagnosis	
• Facilitates rapid diagnosis • Cost-effective • Provides coverage for remote sites • Useful for remote frozen sections • Useful for immediate fine-needle aspiration evaluation • Potential to improve patient care • Load balancing	• Difficult to handle certain cases (eg, multiple simultaneous cases) • Deferral to glass slide may be needed • May take longer than glass slide review • Technology errors and downtime • System maintenance required • State limited licensure
Secondary Consultation	
• Access to expert opinions • Real-time consultation • Cheaper than courier services • Faster turnaround time • Original material retained at host institution • Avoids slide loss or damage • Portability of the telepathologist • Virtual collaboration (teleconferencing)	• Difficult to handle certain cases (eg, cases with multiple slides) • Technical failures • Image quality (especially for difficult cases) • Billing arrangements

improved. However, the interpretation of telecytology digital images is still hindered by the inability of images to accurately display cellular detail (eg, nuclear chromasia) and to change focus along the z-axis, especially in thick areas with overlapping cell groups.

Telepathology has been widely used for intraoperative consultation (eg, frozen section) at a remote location without a pathologist on-site and/or when traveling and/or when shipment of a specimen may be impracticable.[57–59] Most recently, telepathology has started to be used for making primary diagnoses, but this has occurred in countries (eg, Canada) outside the United States. Another area in which telepathology has been extensively used is to facilitate consultation between pathologists.[60,61] Patient-related material (eg, glass slides) may need to be referred for formal secondary review for a number of reasons; that is, expert opinion requested by the primary pathologist for a difficult case, per patient request, or as a result of a patient being referred to another institution for follow-up care. Traditionally, cases (glass slides) are physically sent via commercial courier services. Unfortunately, the risk is that shipped slides may get lost or broken.[62] This risk is virtually eliminated with telepathology, and is particularly helpful when making recut sections is unfeasible or when there are only limited slides available for review.

Telepathology and teleconferencing are ideal for educational purposes.[63] In addition to portability and the ease of sharing cases with multiple users, telepathology ensures consistency and longevity of imaged materials for educational purposes, and offers a mechanism to standardize teaching.[64] An increasing number of teaching programs (eg, medical schools, pathology residency training programs, cytotechnology schools) have created "virtual slide sets" to replace traditional slide boxes. Digital images, linked to case-related information, can be offered online for students anywhere, which can be viewed at any time.[65,66] An increasing number of professional societies and organizations are using WSI for conferencing, continuing medical education, scientific meetings, and proficiency testing.

TELECOMMUNICATION

Telecommunication is the transmission of messages over distances for the purpose of communication. Telepathology is becoming easier to implement in most laboratories, primarily because access to broadband telecommunications and wireless technology is more prevalent.[67] Telepathology systems can be linked to a local area network or wide area network on the Internet via cables, an integrated services digitized network, satellite, or a Wi-Fi connection. The Internet provides universal, simplified, and affordable options for telepathology in most regions. Limitations imposed by the Internet include no guarantees on the quality of service, security and privacy concerns, and for some regions low bandwidth, which negatively impacts real-time applications.[68] Telepathology using wireless telecommunications and mobile phone cellular services has proven to be effective for clinical use.[69,70] Teleconferencing or desktop sharing software (eg, Skype, Lync, Team Viewer), which offers live (synchronous) online communication between distant users, has been used for some telepathology solutions.[71–73] Several online digital sharing services (eg, SecondSlide) have been established. When using a file hosting service (eg, DropBox, PathXchange) for cloud storage and/or file sharing, it is important to make sure that they meet privacy concerns for clinical use, such as the Health Insurance Portability and Accountability Act.

TELEPATHOLOGY MODES AND SYSTEMS

The various modes of telepathology (static, dynamic, WSI, hybrid) are compared in **Table 3**. Static telepathology involves the examination of precaptured still digital

Table 3
Comparison of different telepathology methods

Telepathology Method	Image System	Remote Control	Images Per Case	Image Selection	Bandwidth Needed	Cost
Static	Still	No	Limited	Host	Low	Low
Dynamic	Live	Yes	Unlimited	Telepathologist	High	High
Whole-slide imaging	Still	Yes	Unlimited	Telepathologist	High	High
Hybrid	Still and Live	Yes	Unlimited	Telepathologist	High	High

images (snapshots) that can be transmitted via e-mail or stored on a shared server. Dynamic telepathology involves the examination of live images or a sequence of images in real time using a live telecommunications link. In general, dynamic systems offer greater accuracy because the user can interpret images in real time without limited focus.[74] WSI involves digitization (scanning) of glass slides to produce high-resolution digital slides. Hybrid technology combines robotics with high-resolution imaging.[75–77]

There are several systems available for telepathology. These include gross workstations, microscope cameras, robotic microscopes, and whole-slide scanners. Gross workstations are used primarily to transmit macroscopic images of specimens for gross pathology. Telepathology can be performed using microscopic cameras in 3 ways: (1) static telepathology using a digital camera (or smartphone) attached to a microscope; (2) video microscopy using a video camera connected to a microscope; and (3) teleconferencing where software is used to share the desktop on which a microscopic image is displayed. Early studies using video technology were plagued by slow transmission and poor picture quality.[74,78–81] Robotic telepathology involves remote microscope robotic operation (eg, motorized stage, objectives, and focus). WSI has also been termed wide-field microscopy or "virtual" microscopy. Newer whole-slide scanners now offer remote robotic control to view slides in addition to WSI capabilities.

Static Telepathology

Static (store-and-forward) telepathology can be used to share digital images of just about anything in pathology, such as gross specimens, parasites, microbiology culture plates, histopathology, blood smears, and electrophoresis gels. These images may be shared with others via e-mail or stored on a shared server. The person sending the image and the pathologist receiving it do not need to do so simultaneously (ie, asynchronous telepathology).[82] In addition to still images, other types of information that can be transferred with this technique include audio, text, and video files. Static images can be viewed by a single telepathologist or simultaneously by multiple clients during an online discussion.[83] The benefits of static telepathology are its relatively low cost, simple technology needed, vendor independence, and low maintenance. Moreover, the image files are small and hence easier to manage and store. However, there are several drawbacks, including no remote control access, sampling error, only limited fields of view are available for evaluation, and the host taking the images needs to have some expertise to select appropriate diagnostic fields.[84,85] Static telepathology is typically unsuitable for emergency consultations. Acquiring still images also is labor intensive.

Robotic Telepathology

The first robotic telepathology system was invented and patented by Dr. R.S. Weinstein (Weinstein US Patent #5,216,596). The first patent application was submitted in 1987 and granted in 1993. This form of telepathology involves a robotically controlled microscope with a digital camera attached to the microscope linked to a networked computer. Robotic systems allow one to perform dynamic (real-time) telepathology. The telepathologist has software controls on his or her computer to remotely "drive" (ie, pan and zoom around a slide) and focus the microscope. Advantages of robotic telepathology include access to the entire slide, user control of the microscope and image with respect to fields (panning) and magnification, good image quality, and fast driving speed. In a review of 11 published studies from 1997 to 2007 using robotic telepathology for rendering remote frozen section diagnoses, the diagnostic accuracy ranged between 89% and 100%.[5] Some of the disadvantages include expensive technology, the need for integrated software for both host and recipient, high bandwidth requirements, and the need for ongoing technical support and maintenance.

Whole-Slide Imaging

WSI telepathology offers another means to view an entirely digitized (scanned) slide. Whole-slide scanners typically include a slide loader, microscope with different objectives, digital camera, robotics, and software. Slide loaders range from trays that hold 1 to 4 slides to large racks or hotels that can stack up to 400 slides. For recently mounted slides (eg, frozen section slides with a movable coverslip), it is better to use horizontal loading rather than vertical placement. Slide scanning can be automated or done manually. Slides can be scanned using an objective lens magnification of $\times 20$, $\times 40$, or higher depending on the telepathology need. For routine surgical pathology work, $\times 20$ should suffice; however, for hematopathology cases, $\times 40$ may be preferred, and for telemicrobiology even higher magnification (eg, $\times 83$ oil magnification). The focal plane (orthogonal disposition) also will need to be set before scanning. For cytology cases, z-stacking is often desirable. Although scanning at higher magnification takes longer and results in larger image files, the digital images are of better resolution and offer superior zoom capability. However, large files (eg, 150 GB without compression) require good computer microprocessors and adequate RAM to manipulate them.

WSI has been shown to be remarkably suitable for telepathology, because digital slides are of high resolution and permit access to an entire slide or set of slides at various magnifications.[86,87] Once the scanned slide is ready, viewing the digital image to render a diagnosis can be faster than using a robotic microscope, especially if performed on a computer with a high-speed network connection. The length of time required to prepare slides for scanning and conduct previsualization quality checks should be taken into account when using WSI for rapid telepathology, such as during frozen sections. In one study comparing the time requirements of robotic versus virtual slide telepathology for frozen sections, investigators found that slide preparation time for both modalities was comparable (average 10.33 minutes for robotic vs 12.26 minutes for virtual slides), but that slide interpretation time was far superior with digital slides (average 10.26 minutes for robotic vs 3.42 minutes for virtual slides).[5] Because of the ease related to sharing files and the interactive nature of viewing images, WSI is incredibly effective for education.[88]

At present, WSI telepathology equipment is still expensive for many laboratories. Added expense may be incurred with storage of large image files. With newer scanners, rapid scanning is possible. However, long scan times may result if high-resolution, multiplane images are desired or when digitizing slides with large, thick tissue sections. Scanning difficulties may arise as a result of cover slip misplacement or wet slides with too much mounting medium that stick with automatic slide feeders. Small tissue fragments, faint tissue, or material at the slide edge or even outside the coverslip may not get scanned. For cytopathology, WSI may be problematic without z-stacking. Anther disadvantage of WSI is related to the fact that with some scanners, slides may need to be scanned one at a time. Also, there is currently a lack of vendor interoperability, making it difficult to sometimes view proprietary image files with different viewers.

REFERENCES

1. Weinberg DS. How is telepathology being used to improve patient care? Clin Chem 1996;42:831–5.
2. Weinstein RS, Bhattacharyya AK, Graham AR, et al. Telepathology: a ten-year progress report. Hum Pathol 1997;28:1–7.
3. Kayser K, Szymas J, Weinstein R. Telepathology. Telecommunication, electronic education and publication in pathology. Berlin: Springer; 1999. p. 1–186.
4. Weinstein RS, Graham AR, Richter LC, et al. Overview of telepathology, virtual microscopy, and whole slide imaging: prospects for the future. Hum Pathol 2009;40: 1057–69.
5. Evans AJ, Chetty R, Clarke BA, et al. Primary frozen section diagnosis by robotic microscopy and virtual slide telepathology: the University Health Network experience. Hum Pathol 2009;40:1070–81.
6. Evans AJ, Kiehl TR, Croul S. Frequently asked questions concerning the use of whole-slide imaging telepathology for neuropathology frozen sections. Semin Diagn Pathol 2010;27(3):160–6.
7. Agha Z, Weinstein RS, Dunn BE. Cost minimization analysis of telepathology. Am J Clin Pathol 1999;112:470–8.
8. Kayser K, Beyer M, Blum S, et al. Recent developments and present status of telepathology. Anal Cell Pathol 2000;21:101–6.
9. Weinstein RS, Descour MR, Liang C, et al. Telepathology overview: from concept to implementation. Hum Pathol 2001;32:1283–99.
10. Massone C, Brunasso AM, Campbell TM, et al. State of the art of teledermatopathology. Am J Dermatopathol 2008;30:446–50.
11. Graham AR, Bhattacharyya AK, Scott KM, et al. Virtual slide telepathology for an academic teaching hospital surgical pathology quality assurance program. Hum Pathol 2009;40:1129–36.
12. Lopez AM, Graham AR, Barker GP, et al. Virtual slide telepathology enables an innovative telehealth rapid breast care clinic. Hum Pathol 2009;40:1082–91.
13. Weinstein RS. Prospects for telepathology [editorial]. Hum Pathol 1986;17:433–4.
14. Weinstein RS, Descour MR, Liang C, et al. An array microscope for ultrarapid virtual slide processing and telepathology. Design, fabrication, and validation study. Hum Pathol 2004;35:1303–14.
15. Williams S, Henricks WH, Becich MJ, et al. Telepathology for patient care: what am I getting myself into? Adv Anat Pathol 2010;17:130–49.
16. Kayser K, Szymas J, Weinstein RS. Telepathology and telemedicine: communication, electronic education and publication in e-health. Berlin: VSV Interdisciplinary Medical Publishing; 2005. p. 1–257.

17. Dunn BE, Choi H, Recla DL, et al. Robotic surgical telepathology between the Iron Mountain and Milwaukee Department of Veterans Affairs medical centers: a 12-year experience. Hum Pathol 2009;40:1092–9.

18. Halliday BE, Bhattacharyya AK, Graham AR, et al. Diagnostic accuracy of an international static-imaging telepathology consultation service. Hum Pathol 1997;28:17–21.

19. Nordrum I, Engum B, Rinde E, et al. Remote frozen section service: a telepathology project to northern Norway. Hum Pathol 1991;22:514–8.

20. Kaplan KJ, Burgess JR, Sandberg GD, et al. Use of robotic telepathology for frozen-section diagnosis: a retrospective trial of a telepathology system for intraoperative consultation. Mod Pathol 2002;15:1197–204.

21. O'Malley DP. Practical applications of telepathology using morphology-based anatomic pathology. Arch Pathol Lab Med 2008;132:743–4.

22. Pantanowitz L, Evans AJ, Hassell LA, et al. American Telemedicine Association clinical guidelines for telepathology. J Pathol Inform 2014;5:39.

23. Canadian Association of Pathologists Telepathology Guidelines Committee, Bernard C, Chandrakanth SA, et al. Guidelines from the Canadian Association of Pathologists for establishing a telepathology service for anatomic pathology using whole-slide imaging. J Pathol Inform 2014;28(5):15.

24. Lowe J. Telepathology: guideline from the Royal College of Pathologists. London. 2013. Available at: http://www.rcpath.org/Resources/RCPath/Migrated%20Resources/Documents/G/G026_Telepathology_Oct13.pdf. Accessed March 18, 2015.

25. Leung ST, Kaplan KJ. Medicolegal aspects of telepathology. Hum Pathol 2009; 40:1137–42.

26. Güler NF, Ubeyli ED. Theory and applications of telemedicine. J Med Syst 2002; 26:199–220.

27. Hoyt R, Sutton M, Yoshihashi A. Medical informatics. Practical guide for the healthcare professional. Pensacola (FL): University of West Florida Press; 2007. p. 197–206.

28. Fox BI. Telehealth. In: Felkey BG, Fox BI, Thrower MR, editors. Health care informatics: a skills-based resource. Washington, DC: American Pharmacists Association; 2006. p. 277–300.

29. Stanberry B. Telemedicine: barriers and opportunities in the 21st century. J Intern Med 2000;247:615–28.

30. Picot J. Meeting the need for educational standards in the practice of telemedicine and telehealth. J Telemed Telecare 2000;2(6 Suppl):S59–62.

31. Wells CA, Sowter C. Telepathology: a diagnostic tool for the millennium? J Pathol 2000;191:1–7.

32. Dunn BE, Almagro UA, Choi H, et al. Dynamic-robotic telepathology: Department of Veterans Affairs feasibility study. Hum Pathol 1997;28:8–12.

33. Weinstein RS, Bloom KJ, Rozek LS. Static and dynamic imaging in pathology. IEEE Proc Image Management Comm 1990;1:77–85.

34. Krupinski E, Weinstein RS, Bloom KJ, et al. Progress in telepathology: system implementation and testing. Advances in Path Lab Med 1993;6:63–87.

35. Mullick FG, Fontelo P, Pemble C. Telemedicine and telepathology at the Armed Forces Institute of Pathology: history and current mission. Telemed J 1996;2:187–93.

36. Ongürü O, Celasun B. Intra-hospital use of a telepathology system. Pathol Oncol Res 2000;6:197–201.

37. Ho J, Ahlers SM, Stratman C, et al. Can digital pathology result in cost savings? A financial projection for digital pathology implementation at a large integrated health care organization. J Pathol Inform 2014;5:33.

38. Henricks WH. Evaluation of whole slide imaging for routine surgical pathology: Looking through a broader scope. J Pathol Inform 2012;3:39.
39. Fine JL. 21st century workflow: a proposal. J Pathol Inform 2014;5:44.
40. Brebner EM, Brebner JA, Norman JN, et al. Intercontinental postmortem studies using interactive television. J Telemed Telecare 1997;3:48–52.
41. Fisher SI, Nandedkar MA, Williams BH, et al. Telehematopathology in a clinical consultative practice. Hum Pathol 2001;32:1327–33.
42. McLaughlin WJ, Schifman RB, Ryan KJ, et al. Telemicrobiology: feasibility study. Telemed J 1998;4:11–7.
43. Suhanic W, Crandall I, Pennefather P. An informatics model for guiding assembly of telemicrobiology workstations for malaria collaborative diagnostics using commodity products and open-source software. Malar J 2009;8:164.
44. Schroeder JA. Ultrasrural telepathology: remote EM diagnostic via Internet. In: Kumar S, Dunn BE, editors. Telepathology, vol. 14. Berlin: Springer; 2009. p. 179–204.
45. Yamada A. Remote control of the scanning electron microscope. In: Kumar S, Dunn BE, editors. Telepathology, vol. 15. Berlin: Springer; 2009. p. 205–24.
46. Maiolino P, De Vico G. Telepathology in veterinary diagnostic cytology. In: Kumar S, Dunn BE, editors. Telepathology, vol. 6. Berlin: Springer; 2009. p. 63–70.
47. Pantanowitz L, Hornish M, Goulart RA. The impact of digital imaging in the field of cytopathology. Cytojournal 2009;6:6.
48. Lee ES, Kim IS, Choi JS, et al. Accuracy and reproducibility of telecytology diagnosis of cervical smears. A tool for quality assurance programs. Am J Clin Pathol 2003;119:356–60.
49. Raab SS, Zaleski MS, Thomas PA, et al. Telecytology: diagnostic accuracy in cervical-vaginal smears. Am J Clin Pathol 1996;105:599–603.
50. Schwarzmann P, Schenck U, Binder B, et al. Is today's telepathology equipment also appropriate for telecytology? A pilot study with pap and blood smears. Adv Clin Path 1998;2:176–8.
51. Ziol M, Vacher-Lavenu MC, Heudes D, et al. Expert consultation for cervical carcinoma smears. Reliability of selected-field videomicroscopy. Anal Quant Cytol Histol 1999;21:35–41.
52. Eichhorn JH, Buckner L, Buckner SB, et al. Internet-based gynecologic telecytology with remote automated image selection: results of a first-phase developmental trial. Am J Clin Pathol 2008;129:686–96.
53. Prayaga A. Telecytology: a retrospect and prospect. In: Kumar S, Dunn BE, editors. Telepathology, vol. 12. Berlin: Springer; 2009. p. 149–62.
54. Thrall M, Pantanowitz L, Khalbuss W. Telecytology: clinical applications, current challenges, and future benefits. J Pathol Inform 2011;2:51.
55. Kerr SE, Bellizzi AM, Stelow EB, et al. Initial assessment of fine-needle aspiration specimens by telepathology: validation for use in pathology resident-faculty consultations. Am J Clin Pathol 2008;130:409–13.
56. Allen EA, Ollayos CW, Tellado MV, et al. Characteristics of a telecytology consultation service. Hum Pathol 2001;32:1323–6.
57. Wellnitz U, Binder B, Fritz P, et al. Reliability of telepathology for frozen section service. Anal Cell Pathol 2000;21:213–22.
58. Winokur TS, McClellan S, Siegal GP, et al. A prospective trial of telepathology for intraoperative consultation (frozen sections). Hum Pathol 2000;31:781–5.
59. Liang WY, Hsu CY, Lai CR, et al. Low-cost telepathology system for intraoperative frozen-section consultation: our experience and review of the literature. Hum Pathol 2008;39:56–62.

60. Beltrami CA, Della Mea V. Second opinion consultation through the Internet. A three years experience. Adv Clin Path 1998;2:146–8.
61. Piccolo D, Soyer HP, Burgdorf W, et al. Concordance between telepathologic diagnosis and conventional histopathologic diagnosis: a multiobserver store-and-forward study on 20 skin specimens. Arch Dermatol 2002;138:53–8.
62. Rosen PP. Special report: perils, problems, and minimum requirements in shipping pathology slides. Am J Clin Pathol 1989;91:348–54.
63. Romer DJ, Suster S. Use of virtual microscopy for didactic live-audience presentation in anatomic pathology. Ann Diagn Pathol 2003;7:67–72.
64. Helin H, Lundin M, Lundin J, et al. Web-based virtual microscopy in teaching and standardizing Gleason grading. Hum Pathol 2005;36:381–6.
65. Bruch LA, De Young BR, Kreiter CD, et al. Competency assessment of residents in surgical pathology using virtual microscopy. Hum Pathol 2009;40:1122–8.
66. Dee FR. Virtual microscopy in pathology education. Hum Pathol 2009;40: 1112–21.
67. Alfaro L, Roca MJ. Portable telepathology: methods and tools. Diagn Pathol 2008; 3(Suppl 1):S19.
68. Della Mea V, Beltrami CA. Current experiences with Internet telepathology and possible evolution in the next generation of Internet services. Anal Cell Pathol 2000;21:127–34.
69. Frierson HF Jr, Galgano MT. Frozen-section diagnosis by wireless telepathology and ultra portable computer: use in pathology resident/faculty consultation. Hum Pathol 2007;38:1330–4.
70. Bellina L, Missoni E. Mobile cell-phones (M-phones) in telemicroscopy: increasing connectivity of isolated laboratories. Diagn Pathol 2009;4:19.
71. Marchevsky AM, Lau SK, Khanafshar E, et al. Internet teleconferencing method for telepathology consultations from lung and heart transplant patients. Hum Pathol 2002;33:410–4.
72. McKenna JK, Florell SR. Cost-effective dynamic telepathology in the Mohs surgery laboratory utilizing iChat AV videoconferencing software. Dermatol Surg 2007;33:62–8.
73. Klock C, Gomes Rde P. Web conferencing systems: Skype and MSN in telepathology. Diagn Pathol 2008;3(Suppl 1):S13.
74. Smith MB. Introduction to telepathology. In: Cowan DF, editor. Informatics for the clinical laboratory. A practical guide for the practicing pathologist, vol. 16. New York: Springer; 2005. p. 268–86.
75. Tsuchihashi Y, Mazaki T, Nakasato K, et al. The basic diagnostic approaches used in robotic still-image telepathology. J Telemed Telecare 1999;5(Suppl 1):S115–7.
76. Zhou J, Hogarth MA, Walters RF, et al. Hybrid system for telepathology. Hum Pathol 2000;31:829–33.
77. Della Mea V, Cataldi P, Pertoldi B, et al. Combining dynamic- and static-robotic techniques for real-time telepathology. In: Kumar S, Dunn BE, editors. Telepathology, vol. 8. Berlin: Springer; 2009. p. 79–89.
78. Callas PW, Leslie KO, Mattia AR, et al. Diagnostic accuracy of a rural live video telepathology system. Am J Surg Pathol 1997;21:812–9.
79. Baak JP, van Diest PJ, Meijer GA. Experience with a dynamic inexpensive video-conferencing system for frozen section telepathology. Anal Cell Pathol 2000;21: 169–75.
80. Prasse KW, Mahaffey EA, Duncan JR, et al. Accuracy of interpretation of microscopic images of cytologic, hematologic, and histologic specimens using a low-resolution desktop video conferencing system. Telemed J 1996;2:259–66.

81. Vazir MH, Loane MA, Wootton R. A pilot study of low-cost dynamic telepathology using the public telephone network. J Telemed Telecare 1998;4:168–71.
82. Della Mea V. Prerecorded telemedicine. J Telemed Telecare 2005;11:276–84.
83. Brauchli K, Oberli H, Hurwitz N, et al. Diagnostic telepathology: long-term experience of a single institution. Virchows Arch 2004;444:403–9.
84. Della Mea V, Cataldi P, Boi S, et al. Image selection in static telepathology through the Internet. J Telemed Telecare 1998;4(Suppl 1):20–2.
85. Della Mea V, Cataldi P, Boi S, et al. Image sampling in static telepathology for frozen section diagnosis. J Clin Pathol 1999;52:761–5.
86. Wilbur DC, Madi K, Colvin RB, et al. Whole-slide imaging digital pathology as a platform for teleconsultation: a pilot study using paired subspecialist correlations. Arch Pathol Lab Med 2009;133:1949–53.
87. Furness P. A randomized controlled trial of the diagnostic accuracy of Internet-based telepathology compared with conventional microscopy. Histopathology 2007;50:266–73.
88. Góngora Jará H, Barcelo HA. Telepathology and continuous education: important tools for pathologists of developing countries. Diagn Pathol 2008;3(Suppl 1):S24.

Selection and Implementation of New Information Systems

 CrossMark

Keith J. Kaplan, MD[a],*, Luigi K.F. Rao, MD, MS[b]

KEYWORDS

- Laboratory information system • Implementation • Selection • Workflow

OVERVIEW: SELECTION
Background and Concepts

Do I really need a new system? How do I go about that process? Do I want to replace what I have? Is what I have good enough, so that all I need to do is surround it with additional capabilities?

How do you go about finding out which candidates are the correct systems for you? Do you want to go best of breed, or do you want to have a single vendor?

Regardless of your current practice—its members, partners, hospitals, and laboratories that comprise your practice—these questions are almost always the same.

Workflow can be broadly defined as an orchestrated and repeatable pattern of business activity enabled by the systematic organization of resources into processes that transform materials, provide services, or process information.[1]

The single most important element to consider when evaluating clinical information systems for your practice is workflow.[2] You want your anatomic pathology (AP) laboratory information system (LIS) to fit your existing workflows or improve them but not redesign them to meet the requirements of the LIS. Software can be modified to meet your physical and virtual needs much easier than the converse. Many people make the mistake of evaluating the features of the software and all that they can and perhaps initially cannot do as areas for improvement and lose sight of how any of them fit into existing operations and desired workflows. Although many of the particular functions of the software may change or be modified as you customize the features, the particular workflows of your laboratory, perhaps on its third or fourth LIS system, are unlikely to change as often. Workflows within laboratories, ideally, are designed over time with particular goals or deliverables in mind and exist and persist to meet

This article originally appeared in Surgical Pathology Clinics, Volume 8, Issue 2, June 2015.
Dr K.J. Kaplan is the Publisher for www.tissuepathology.com.
[a] PO Box 473431, Charlotte, NC 28247, USA; [b] Department of Pathology, Walter Reed National Military Medical Center, 8901 Rockville Pike, Bethesda, MD 20889, USA
* Corresponding author.
E-mail address: keithjkaplanmd@gmail.com

those goals after years of refinements. Although they may not seem ideal to an outsider, they may be completely practical and functional in an established laboratory to meet its specific needs with its patients, providers, technical staff, partner laboratories and/or hospitals, vendors, clients, and customers. An information system without your workflow in mind will not achieve the overall goals of any implementation—increased efficiency, increased productivity, and cost savings with measurable return on investment (ROI).

Practical matters, such as accessioning, gross processing, histology processing, workload assignment, case distribution, additional test ordering, case resulting, and result delivery, may seem like routine, mundane, basic requirements of any AP LIS; however, you may find particular vendors' thoughts on laboratory workflow may not fit yours. They may not appreciate assigning certain cases to certain pathologists perhaps at the time of accessioning based on client requirements rather than at case assembly as many laboratories have historically done. Conversely, you may not want cases assigned at accessioning but perhaps the following day when slides are cut and stained, the daily schedule is known, and the volume of cases, blocks, slides, and staffing are up to the minute.

Without getting too far ahead in the overall evaluation process, the most practical way to do this is to process a week's worth of specimens through a mock installation in tandem with your soon-to-be legacy system and see how one compares with the other, focusing not on "how" the system may necessarily perform a certain task but asking "why" does the system behave in this fashion. What rules, logic, recent enhancements/upgrades, or potential opportunities or issues upstream or downstream from that process may be affected for the next user in the process? For example, what may look like a nice shortcut or feature at accessioning may look attractive; if it creates potential for error at grossing, embedding, or with the immunohistochemistry stainer interface, you need to address the pain points early in the process to ensure workflow requirements are met for all users.

With that said, it cannot be assumed that a prospective LIS does something in a manner that is different from how you currently handle a portion of your workflow or that the new LIS, or at least that part of it, is inferior to your current system. Commercially available systems often represent an aggregate of workflow solutions that have been validated by current customers with enhancements provided in the form of upgrades to the current versioning of the application. Thus, much as new information is learned when conducting peer reviews of other laboratories and often new workflows are implemented based on experience elsewhere, the proposed solution in terms of a new LIS may offer some functionality that would be an improvement to your existing workflow but perhaps unable to perform due to current system limitations and workarounds put in place many years ago that have become routine workflow without anyone able to recall, "Why it is we do it this way?" other than the tried and true explanation, "That is the way we have always done it."

Vendors may make claims that their system supports your particular workflow or portion thereof that is of concern while perhaps not having done so before but would be willing to provide that specification as a customization to their existing system. In general, instead of implementing their current solution in your laboratory for a week, as previously discussed, to detail what level of customization to their source code is required to meet an important detail of your workflow, which is impractical, speak with current customers or references provided by the LIS vendor. Ideally you may know of or be provided a list of clients who use the software currently that are similar in scope and volume to your laboratory.

References are an economical source of valuable information, whether their experience has been overall positive or negative with the application. Most speak openly about a company, product, implementation, validation, testing, production, and ongoing service, support, and upgrades. Here you can uncover issues related to the performance of the company, the application, installation, or post go-live issues that another laboratory has experienced. Be prepared with a list of questions that address their experience today with a particular vendor and application. You may not need this list if you have a talkative reference, but it will help organize an important part of your due diligence in this process. Address workflow and any current or previous issues they had or uncovered that may be an issue for your operation. Also address any customizations that were or were not supported to address those concerns. Customization is a complex process that involves both the laboratory and the vendor to complete successfully. Hearing from another laboratory that it was or was not a pleasant experience may go a long way in your decision making. Be sure to address what resources they had internally to work with the vendor and what resource the vendor supplied to the project and balance those with your resources, or lack thereof, if you have the skills, support, and time to work with the vendor on developing.

Selection

Armed with a basic concept of how to approach system requirements within your laboratory's environment and workflow considerations and a decision made to explore and potentially select a new AP LIS, consider a request for information or request for proposal (RFI/RFP) from vendors to respond to for potential selection. Many companies, such as the College of American Pathologists and KLAS, regularly provide lists of commercially available LIS systems and ratings, respectively, to begin to research companies and products. Although much of the information is self-reported, both sources of information provide a common starting point for many to begin your own research.

A common starting point is to submit an RFI/RFP to vendors you think may be suitable based on install base, size and scope of clients, interface experience, previous experience, and customer feedback. This initial filter is important only in terms of considering how many companies you would like to potentially demonstrate their system for you, site visits to attend, and reference calls to make initially. You may want to choose from a wide range of small and large companies with any AP experience or limit the range. This commitment likely is long-term one for your laboratory, so be sure to address whether a particular product has been in use for several years at multiple locations and the likelihood it will continue to be so for years to come. What are the mission and vision for a company and its applications? Do they align with your core business model and practices?

The RFI/RFP may go a long way in terms of vendors selected for the next phase or eliminated from consideration based on their responses.

A couple of sample, high-level RFI/RFP approaches are provided in different forms to consider using as a road map for your own organization based on its specific needs and requirements. Some of these may not apply or be a short- or long-term consideration. At this phase, it may not hurt to ask about a company's thoughts on a particular specification should that need become necessary in a few months to years, perhaps during the time an implementation may be started or is finishing. The laboratory business is constantly changing and information technology (IT) needs to be fluid to respond to those changes and paramount to these are AP LIS performance issues even if they do seem like a "nice to have" but not a "must have" today.

Sample Request for Information or Request for Proposal #1
Technical environment
Hardware

Describe the required hardware configuration, including descriptions of central processing unit(s), networking hardware, back-up devices, and uninterruptible power supply.

Describe the ability of the proposed system to support fail-safe data storage (redundancy, mirrored, and so forth).

Describe the requirements of system cabling for communication to the server and to the existing network.

Does the system employ 32-bit architecture?

What are the warranty periods provided for hardware?

Please outline service and maintenance costs for the system as proposed.

In an outreach environment, describe the connectivity of the proposed system.

Software

Describe the operating systems under which the proposed system will operate (UNIX, DOS, Windows, Windows NT, and so forth).

Name and describe the database management program utilized by the system.

What programming language(s) was used to develop the system?

Describe the file purging/archiving methodology used by the proposed system.

List cost of license agreements, renewal, and upgrades.

Describe the length of time a software version is supported.

Please describe your system's database reporting tools.

Describe the security system used by the proposed system.

Describe your proposed disaster recovery plan to safeguard source code and ensure that the proposed system is recoverable in the event of a disaster at the headquarters of your facility.

Describe your proposed disaster recovery plan to ensure that data are safe and secure in the event of a disaster.

Network and interface issues

Have you interfaced your LIS with other clinical information systems? (Provide names of interfaced systems.)

Describe the network topology of your outreach solution in conjunction with your LIS solution.

Describe the network topology of your outreach solution in conjunction with another vendor's LIS solution.

Can your outreach solution be a stand-alone application utilizing a different LIS?

Have you interfaced your outreach solution with other information systems (ie, the outreach solution needs to be able to accept orders from and send results to information systems that do not reside on the same local area network [LAN] or wide area network [WAN] as the laboratory)?

Does the proposed system comply with Health Level Seven International interface standards for importing and exporting data to and from other systems?

Have you interfaced your LIS with reference laboratories? (Provide names of interface reference laboratories.) Describe the interface functionality.

Does your LIS have the capability to provide a direct link to off-site locations for order entry and result retrieval? Describe this capability in detail.

What communication protocols are supported?

What speeds of network lines are required for proposed LIS to function on WAN?

What network infrastructure is needed to operate a true outreach operation (ie, the laboratory needs to accept orders from and send results to a nursing home that is not within the same LAN or WAN as the laboratory)?

SYSTEM IMPLEMENTATION AND TECHNICAL SUPPORT

Describe and attach your typical implementation plan. Describe the length of time your engineer will be on site during implementation and the exact scope of the work he/she will perform.

Describe the experience and qualifications of your installation team.

What kind of client communication and implementation planning is done prior to the installation?

Describe the training provided. Include a training outline.

Where is your technical support center located?

What are the methods for contacting technical support?

What are your hours of operation for technical support?

Describe the qualifications of your technical support staff.

Describe the organization and structure of your technical support services.

What percentage of your total employees is responsible for direct client support?

Describe the ongoing system support provided by the vendor.

Are software upgrades provided as part of the software support contract?

Describe your software upgrade process.

Are there "hot fixes" or "updates" between versions? Do these updates cost extra?

How often are new versions released?

How are customer requests for enhancements and customizations handled?

How many separate modifications were included in the last release?

How many separate modifications included in the last release requested by current users?

Describe the qualifications of your product development department.

What percentage of your total employees is responsible for product development?

Do you have a formal users' group?

Describe the company's policy regarding source code.

System Proposal

Provide a system proposal that includes

- Detailed listing of hardware provided
- Detailed listing of software provided
- Description of training provided, including location and time commitment
- Description and cost of ongoing support
- Cost of proposed system

Sample Request for Information or Request for Proposal #2

List of functional requirements Assign one of the following availability codes to each item:

A—Feature is available off the shelf.

N—Feature is not available.

C—Feature is available with additional cost and custom programming.

- Detailed responses to and descriptions of each checklist item mentioned are required.
- Elaborate on any items that differentiate you from other vendors.

- Failure to complete or respond to all checklist items may result in dismissal of your RFI/RFP submission. If you do not have the functionality mentioned, please respond accordingly with "not available," "in development" or "in testing" or if you would propose doing so at additional cost and customization following the appropriate code (C).

Technical requirements

Describe hardware requirements (see previous example questions).

Describe software requirements (see previous example questions).

Describe network and interface issues (see previous example questions).

Interfacing

Provide operational interfaces for the following applications:
- Hospital information system (HIS)
- Reference laboratory
- Electronic medical record (EMR)
- Billing system
- Practice management system
- Demographics system
- Pathology module/software
- Microbiology module/software
- Radiology module/software
- Other information system(s)

Provide additional interfaces for multiple systems

Provide all interfaces as an integral part of the application requiring no additional third-party software to implement or maintain the interface.

Provide technical support for all active interfaces.

Provide operational interfaces for the following applications (please provide a functional description of each interface available):

HIS

Reference laboratory

EMR

LIS

Billing system

Practice management system

Demographics system

Pathology module/software

Microbiology module/software

Radiology module/software

Other information system

Provide additional interfaces for multiple systems.

Provide all interfaces as an integral part of the application requiring no additional third-party software to implement or maintain the interface.

Provide technical support for all active interfaces.

Security and auditing

Provide a multilevel security system that is separate from the LIS to ensure the confidentiality of patient-related information and to control access to outreach functions and features.

Restrict access to specific areas of the application based on system function to be performed.

Provide practice level security ensuring that associates of one practice cannot gain access to the patient records of another practice.

Allow password protection at different levels (system administrator, phlebotomy, nursing, provider, and so forth).

Allow a user of proper security clearance to modify the database parameters once the system is live, without requiring programming knowledge.

Restrict access to configuration tables, profile indexes, and so forth to designated personnel via security controls.

Maintain an automated system log of user sign-on activity.

Maintain an audit trail for system entries, including user code, date, and time of each system transaction.

Provide multilevel password security down to options within menus.

Provide a multilevel security system that is separate from the LIS to ensure the confidentiality of patient-related information and to control access to outreach functions and features.

Restrict access to specific areas of the application based on system function to be performed.

Provide practice level security ensuring that associates of one practice cannot gain access to the patient records of another practice.

Allow password protection at different levels (system administrator, phlebotomy, nursing, provider, and so forth).

Allow a user of proper security clearance to modify the database parameters once the system is live, without requiring programming knowledge.

Restrict access to configuration tables, profile indexes, and so forth to designated personnel via security controls.

Maintain an automated system log of user sign-on activity.

Maintain an audit trail for system entries including user code, date, and time of each system transaction.

Provide multilevel password security down to options within menus.

Order entry

Allow multiple tests ordering for a single patient using a common demographic record.

Allow laboratory orders to be entered from any computer on or off the local network.

Allow the laboratory to develop and customize orderable items.

Allow simple test ordering: single header linked to a single test result field (eg, glucose).

Allow compound test ordering: single header linked to multiple test result fields (eg, complete blood cell count [CBC], lipid panel, and comprehensive metabolic panel).

Allow the user to order tests by entering test codes and/or by selecting from a test menu.

Automatically alerts users to previously ordered laboratory work.

Allow at the time of ordering a request that patient laboratory results be sent to more than one provider.

Allow the cancellation of orders for patients who do not show for appointment.

Provide medical necessity validation based on laboratory-defined valid diagnosis codes for each applicable test.

Allow the generation of Medicare-compliant Advanced Beneficiary Notice forms when test ordering fails medical necessity validation.

Allow entry of 4 diagnosis codes for each ordered test.

Provide automatic testing destination routing as specified in payor's contract.

Provide automatic label printing as orders are entered.

Allow laboratory-defined label configuration.

Describe the bar code formats your outreach solution accepts and prints.

Provide the specific sample requirements or sample tube types at the time of order entry.

Store diagnosis codes in registration function.

Support retrieval of patient records by partial (eg, first few letters of) patient last name.

Support sample storage and retrieval modules for the purpose of drug testing, add-on testing, and so forth.

Process orders for profiles that include multiple tests (eg, cardiac enzyme profile).

Allow a miscellaneous test code so previously undefined tests can be ordered and charged.

Ability to correct a field on a screen without having to re-enter entire order transaction.

Allow splitting one ordered test into more than one request (eg, group tests, pre-operative, and coagulation screen).

Automatically check for and warn of duplicate single test orders with profile orders.

Support cancellation of tests—logging accession number, test code, patient name, reason, date, time, and tech ID.

Provide simple method to order additional test requests on sample already received and processed in laboratory.

Allow cancellation of an order without canceling prior results.

Provide flexible, customizable sample ID formats.

Print sample collection labels for timed and routine collections.

Allow for multiple labels per test to print.

Print instructions/comments (eg, do not collect from right arm) on sample labels.

Print aliquot labels when more than one test is drawn in the same collection tube.

Provide that uncollected samples continue to appear on subsequent lists until canceled or collected.

Provide for easy free text entry of information, such as critical result notification, sample rejection, or culture sites.

Provide for intelligent prompting for accessioning (eg, when a wound culture is ordered, the system prompts the user for site/location).

Provide easy access to sample requirements for laboratory users.

Provide intelligent sample labeling—groups samples in chemistry together and prints on labels, while hematology tests print on separate label and microbiology prints separately. Allows for making the number of labels customizable for each test.

Provide intuitive user interface—easy to locate screens for accessioning, reporting queries, and so forth.

Provide for an easy, systematic, and logical method of adding, editing, or deleting tests in the test code dictionary.

When looking up a patient in the system, tests performed on that patient and test results are made available without additional steps.

Allow outreach clients to customize their own order entry screens to fit their practice's needs.

Allow outreach clients to customize colors and logos of the system for their practice only.

Result reporting

Provide ability to auto deliver results by the following methods:

Web delivered (ie, provider logs in to a Web site to retrieve results)

E-mail

Fax

Print

Electronic interface to client information system (EMR, HIS, medical practice management software, and so forth)

Accept images, graphics, and linked documents from a host LIS via interface to display on reports.

Provide ability to designate HTML or PDF format of reports.

Maintain patient result history indefinitely.

Provide ability to purge results after a specific amount of time if desired.

Provide ability to graph historical results on a report.

Provide scheduler for automatic result delivery.

Allow redelivery of results.

Automatically maintain a record of reports delivered by each reporting modality (fax, printer, and e-mail, and so forth). Provide easy access to these results at any time.

Allow patient test to be incomplete for at least 8 weeks in the system.

Print daily detailed master log of all work performed in laboratory for audit purposes.

Display abnormal or critical results uniquely from other results.

Allow for cumulative result reporting. Please explain.

Describe the procedure for correcting test results that have been resulted. After correcting, are the corrections able to be altered?

Print list of received but untested samples due to insufficient quantity.

Allow for a comment to be placed on the sample accordingly.

Includes features that allow batch reporting.

Allow features for customizable patient report formats.

Display patient results in an easy to view format for all patients of a provider or location.

Provide ability to batch print and batch acknowledge receipt of results.

Provide the date/time reported on reports transmitted by fax, laser printer, and e-mail.

Provide a permanent log of all test results that have been edited.

Workstations work independently of each other. Multiple functions can occur simultaneously without one party having to exit the system.

Provide flexible reporting formats.

Provide the ability to access all patients of a particular client by name, date, or date range.

Allow look-up of patient and patient results by client number.

Rules-based logic

Ability for rules-based logic where laboratory personnel can define criteria in "if-then" statements.

Ability for rules program to evaluate all rule entries for tests, not just the first one, so that complex or "cascading" rules may easily be designed, where several rules can be invoked based on one scenario.

Provide rules-based report routing.

Provide the ability to create rules to assist in decision support.

Must have ability to flag results based on criteria other than standard reference ranges to include testing location, drawing location, ordering provider, patient age, and priority of order.

Charge rule capability.

Provide ability to customize order entry rules.

Allow rules to be enabled by practice (ie, one practice has certain rules enabled and another practice does not).

Sample status and tracking

Provide the ability to track patient samples throughout the testing process.

Provide identification (ID) of the individual who ordered the test, collected the sample, and released the test results, including the date and time of these occurrences so that this information is accessible throughout the process.

Support user-defined priorities.

Support a way to identify the phlebotomist (doctor, nurse, and so forth) in system for samples not drawn by laboratory personnel.

Include data for tracing order (dates, times, tech ID, and results) from order entry to final reporting in master log.

Provide index to master log by accession number.

Provide customizable sample storage tracking, including ID of freezers, refrigerators, and so forth.

Allow sample storage/retrieval by use of a barcode scanner (ie, the requisition is scanned into the system and the system tells the laboratory where the sample is stored in the laboratory).

Management and administration

Provide ability to create completion reports by date.

Provide ability to create billing summary reports by date.

Provide ability to create reports of failed medical necessity checks.

Provide ability to create canceled test reports that include test name and reason for cancellation.

Provide for a customizable overdue report that would indicate tests, such as urine cultures, that become overdue at 4 days while blood cultures become overdue at 7 days and CBC overdue at 4 hours.

Provide ability to create turnaround time reports by date.

Provide a summary report for test usage over a user-definable period of time.

Provide physician utilization report (eg, number of tests requested by a physician).

Provide ability to print a list of draws that need to be performed.

Patient records

Provide ability to easily generate historical patient reports.

Allow patient database search based on

Patient name

Patient account number

Patient Social Security number

Allow the user to search previous patient results for specific tests and easily view historical results of that test.

Allow the user to graph patient results by test to identify possible trends.

Allow historical results for multiple tests to be graphed on one normalized graph.

Describe how the system handles storage of old results. Is archiving/purging necessary?

Allow the user to review specific patient's results without paging through the entire list of patient results.

Data mining

Provide user-friendly report generator with graphic user interface as an integral part of the outreach application.

Provide ability to create reports from any computer.

Provide ability to create a billing report.

Provide ability to create a report showing all tests completed during a date range.

Provide ability to create a report for order exceptions.

Provide ability to generate patient lists (with certain demographic data) that meet specific result criteria for public health reporting.

Provide ability to create reports on standing or recurring orders.

Provide ability to write queries using logic in great detail within the application.

Support the use of commercially available tools for report generation.

Provide ability to save commonly performed searches.

Provide ability to schedule automatic, unattended runs of data reports.

Provide ability to create reports to mine patient data for specific practices within the application.

Provide online help screens to assist novice users in all applications.

After responses to the RFI/RFP (**Table 1**) customized from the options and others, you may want to include for your laboratory get cost quotations for the system according to your requirements. Be sure to look at initial implementation costs as well as costs for the following 1-, 3-, and 5-year periods for total cost of ownership with ongoing support and maintenance as well as depreciation on the hardware for the total cost of the system to gain a full measure of ROI. Again, at this point, telephone reference checks are an economical way to talk with your peers about the system you are considering.[3]

Once you have narrowed down the possible list of candidate systems to choose from, it is time for vendor demonstrations. Demonstrations are extremely important. If you are going to have 2 or 3 vendors come in, have them come in at the same time or as close to it possible. You have an opportunity to go from one vendor to the other, see something at the first vendor, then go to the second vendor and see if that vendor has it as well. Also, if you spread demonstrations out over time, people are going to forget what they saw. Be sure to include as many shareholders/stakeholders in the process as possible. This is a critical time for someone in accessioning or billing or for a pathologist to question something seen, or more importantly not seen, or that the company was not able to address clearly, to raise concerns about workflow functionality.

Understand your vendor's business strategy. Where are they going? What market are they after? If you are a midsize reference laboratory, for example, and the vendor's primary target market is large academic teaching hospitals, you need to consider the consequences. Also, what do you need to do to install and keep the system running? If you cannot have a medical technologist who is fairly up on IT components and can write the expert rules, and you have to hire 3 programmers to do that, that is something you have to understand.

This visit is also important for understanding the basic architecture of the system and what operating system the system runs on, which are important in the context of other laboratory software applications for functionality as well as those of any corporate partners, hospitals, or clients.

Be cognizant of site visit(s) and users' opinions of the system from due diligence through contracting, implementation, validation, testing, go-live, post–go-live support, and maintenance/upgrades since go-live. Be sure that knowledgeable IT, technical, and professional personnel are available to discuss the pros and cons with you openly. The vendor should not be present at these discussions to allow the client to be completely transparent with their opinions about the company and product. Make a concerted effort to follow specimens from collection to sign-out to see all components of the system. If billing or result interfaces are required or desired, be sure to inquire what systems their LIS interfaces with and their experiences. A site with multiple users/customers who express serious doubts about the company and/or product may be a red flag. Although no system can be everything to everyone, a current user who expresses nothing but frustration with the company and/or the product and regrets either implementing a solution or migrating from a previous solution needs to be addressed in your due diligence. It may be that a customer's expectations were not met based on functionality that did not exist or it may be that a customer was misled by the vendor, as discussed previously. This needs to be sorted out.

Although vendors have different strengths and weaknesses, the aggregate — the area under the end of the curve in integral calculus — for most of the leading vendors is about the same. What is different is how we/they do certain things.[3]

It is also worthwhile to make the time and necessary budget to visit a vendor's headquarters during this process and meet with leadership and see how the customer

Table 1
Sample request for information or request for proposal #3

Enterprise Features	Required/ Desired Optional	Score
Multisite capability?		
Sign-out via Web interface? (No need for VPN, Citrix, or terminal server?)		
Clinical pathology system included		
Build our own interfaces to clients, EMRs, instruments, etc., without vendor fees or involvement?		
Subtotal		
Scalability		
Can system accommodate current volumes?		
Can system accommodate 100% increase to current volumes?		
Database supports mirroring/replication failover?		
Experience configuring and supporting mirrored/replicated environments?		
Subtotal		
System set-up and accession		
Build our own part types?		
Field to store office chart number?		
Mini vs maxi accessioning capability?		
Custom data entry screens by site? Specimen type?		
Enter both AP and clinical data?		
Configurable workflows?		
Custom report generation without vendor assistance?		
Subtotal		
Histology production		
Dynamic notification of special stain and recut orders? E-mail notification?		
Automated logs? Print on defined schedule?		
Subtotal		
Outreach tools		
Interface to practice management systems?		
Result interfaces for common EMRs and hospital systems?		
Autofax/fax on demand?		
Fax chutes by location, client, physician?		
Real-time numeric and graphic client data tracking volume, etc.?		
Custom client productivity reports?		
Subtotal		
Interface capabilities		
Interfaces to Aperio?		
Interfaces to stainer(s)?		
Interfaces to slide and cassette printers?		

(continued on next page)

Table 1
(continued)

Enterprise Features	Required/ Desired Optional	Score
Support for scanned supporting documentation (Reqs, Ins, send-out reports, etc.?)		
Import slide images remotely via Citrix or terminal server?		
Subtotal		
Paperless solutions		
Ability to scan documents in?		
Bar coding?		
RFID?		
Launch case automatically on screen with gross description/ preliminary transcription, attached scan of req, prompted by slide bar code/RFID detection?		
Subtotal		
Transcription productivity		
Quick text templates?		
Medical spell check?		
Synoptic reports (CAP-approved cancer reporting)?		
Means to designate cancer registry reports?		
WYSIWYG throughout report generation?		
Subtotal		
Sign-out		
Ability to easily navigate from module to module without need to exit one or the other?		
Do quick searches?		
Check on history?		
Ability to know if a pathologist has referred the case to another pathologist?		
Transmit e-mail to pathologist that case is transcribed (for rush or other critical cases)?		
One-click sign out? (Cases automatically move to the next in line after sign out.)		
Subtotal		
Vendor qualifications		
Other software products that could be integrated with these products are available.		
Active user group exists for each product.		
User group influences release of the product (eg, controls x% of enhancements to the product).		
Reference sites provided for each product		
Published evaluations of software provided		
Proof of success in similar organization provided		
Willing to demonstrate products: at customer site; at vendor site		
Proposed contract provided		

(continued on next page)

Table 1 (continued)		
Enterprise Features	Required/ Desired Optional	Score
Sample plans provided (eg, implementation, training)		
Software license agreements provided (eg, software maintenance, support)		
Subtotal		
Warranty/support		
Documentation updated for any fixes		
Procedures for vendor-initiated fixes provided		
On-site expertise available at no or low cost		
Customer can modify software without impacting warranty or support		
Updates, enhancements, and new releases covered under maintenance agreements		
Failure to install an update, enhancement, or new release impacts the warranty/support/maintenance after		
30 d or Less		
31–60 d		
61–90 d		
91+ d		
Warranty/support/maintenance is provided for modifications specifically requested by the customer.		
Subtotal		
Total score		

Abbreviations: Reqs, requisitions; RFID, radio frequency identification; VPN, virtual private network; WYSIWYG, what you see is what you get.

service center operates and what the corporate culture is like. Now is the time to know if it has a full-functional 24/7 help desk within the headquarters or whether it outsources that service and how that is managed. One question we like to ask at the headquarter visit of the chief executive officer or chief operating officer is, "What are 3 items you are working on now?" or "What 3 major functionalities do you see on the short-term horizon of importance to clinical laboratories?" Meet the people who are going to be installing and supporting your system. You are going to be business associates and colleagues for potentially the next 7 to 10 years.

Scenarios to provide each vendor may be helpful so that you can compare how one system does a specific function to another. For example, have 10 to 15 scenarios for them to demonstrate, such as assigning specific cases to specific pathologists based on client requests, processing reflex testing, preordering special stain requests, and running a report for client services on volumes of orders/tests received as a month-to-month comparison for business analytics. Ensure that the demonstrations and site visits are the current version and not "mocked up" with functionality that does not exist in a production environment or a database that is unrealistic for clinical use with missing patient identifiers or generic specimen sources, types, or procedures. Try to have the team get some hands-on exposure, to the extent possible, during demonstrations and perhaps on the site visit(s) interact with the system enough to get a flavor of working with the system. You and your laboratory will be seeing this wallpaper on their computer screens for some time.

Folks who are part of the due diligence process need to record and share their thoughts at every stage of the process in the event it is later discovered that part of the RFI/RFP, responses, demonstration, or site visit was incomplete, and that they need to go back to and ensure the specification or functionality was discussed as to whether the system has the capability or not and how it is currently used in a similar clinical environment, if at all.

When multiple vendors are on site at the same time, you have a chance to revisit these vendors, confirm things, and fill in the gaps. If you see a demonstration of one component from one vendor and 2 hours later see the same demonstration from another vendor and see something they are doing that is totally different, go back and ask the first vendor, "Show me how you could do that same function."[3]

Lastly, make a decision and stick to it. You are entering into a long-term relationship most likely, so time is required to make the right decision but the decision-making process should not take longer than it will to implement and validate the system for use, in general. Begin the process of contracting with 4 major principles in mind[3]:

1. The worst time to negotiate a contract is during contract negotiations. You have lost leverage if you have told the vendor they are your choice over all the others.
2. There are standard contracts that are presented. These are a good baseline but the final version may not resemble the original boilerplate version you were initially presented. Often there is good infrastructure there with which to work that you can build on.
3. The contract has to cover the entire system. If you are acquiring hardware, software, implementation services, support, database training, user training, and more, the contract should cover it all.
4. The contract has to be fair and protect the interests of both parties. Without going into an exhaustive review of types of contracts and stipulations within contracts, the reader should recognize legal counsel should be sought for assistance in contract matters of this complexity.

Have a negotiation team prior to contracting. If you want the first year of on-site support to be included beginning at go-live, be sure to include this in negotiations or better yet within the RFI/RFP as a requirement. This is important (discussed later). The vendor may agree to include support but it may affect the price inclusive at implementation rather than an optional line item in the contract. Both sides need to be flexible and not adversarial. Again, the intent is a long-term relationship that requires the terms of the relationship are clearly delineated on the front end. Being treated poorly before you are a client during this process may present some additional information as to whether you want to associate your business with theirs.

A contract checklist should include, but may not be limited to, the following items[3]:

1. System specifications
2. Operational characteristics, including performance criteria, reliability and availability criteria, and backup and recovery
3. Acceptance testing criteria. Make installment payments for capital expenses and implementation based on milestones the vendor has to achieve to be remunerated. For example, you may want to propose 20% of purchase price due at signing, 20% due at database configuration, 15% due at validation, 15% due at

testing, 10% due at go-live, and 20% due at 60 or 90 days post–go-live to resolve any bugs that are identified.
4. Terms and conditions of the license. How much are additional licenses and how few can be purchased at 1 time?
5. Payment terms (discussed previously)
6. Source code availability and user programming provisions and constraints. If the vendor goes out of business, you have the right to find some fallback procedure, whether it is access to source code or the ability to hire a third party to maintain the system for you.
7. Warranties
8. Inclusion of RFI/RFP responses. It is important that they respond to the RFI/RFP in a manner that reflects they meet a particular requirement that was demonstrated and that the production version satisfies the response and demonstration.
9. Confidentiality of data
10. Provisions for additional locations
11. Rights to future applications
12. Manuals and other documentation
13. Legal conditions and remedies. Consult an attorney.

If all goes right, you will have selected the best system to meet your needs within your workflows, to add efficiencies, productivity, and data mining capabilities for both clinical and operational business considerations with a measurable ROI. And in 7 to 10 years' time you may want to do it all over again!

SYSTEM IMPLEMENTATION

Now that the critical aspects of selection of a new information system are covered, focus shifts to implementing this designated system. Although your institution-specific considerations will drive many of the significant decisions surrounding whether to use your chosen vendor's standard functionality or configure for your own environment, the general principles highlighted cover many possible scenarios. And although the discussion remains focused on AP, the overarching themes of the criticality of workflow considerations, a team-centric approach, and multiple iterations of testing remain the same in meeting the needs of implementing a clinical pathology or digital imaging system (among other potential applications).

It would be remiss to not mention the implications of the widespread adoption of electronic health records on the LIS arena,[4] particularly as EHR vendors begin to encroach into space that historically was the lone domain of LIS companies. These developments have often compelled LIS managers and their teams to take on a more involved role, and such involvement needs to be considered because personnel time commitments and expectations rapidly change in this type of scenario. Such considerations are particularly worth dedicating thought and time to if your practice and associated IT support are small in size and/or perhaps larger with more resources and personnel but geographically spread across a large swath of area. Should your technical group be limited in either number, time, and/or adaptability, utilizing a contractor, either wrapped within the original contract with your vendor or as a third-party consultant, may be worthwhile, especially if it offers expertise and seasoned experience as a broker for both sides (of course not losing sight of this temporary but not insignificant expense). Regardless of which approach is taken, a project manager ultimately responsible for the implementation's success should be designated to guide the team through the overall process to completion.

Preparation Phase

In the preparation phase, it is essential to ensure that you and your working environment have made any necessary upgrades to hardware (including computer workstations, servers, printers, and ports) required to take on the new information system. Along the same vein, ensuring that your bandwidth capacity can withstand the demands of the new network requirements is also of prime importance, especially in the context of your institutional security parameters.

Your data conversion and contingency plans are of paramount significance because they will cover which data are carried forward, how the data elements are moved, and by which means legacy data will be accessible while migrated to your new system. Depending on your institution's requirements, you may not feel the need for comprehensive coverage but expect to ask for total 100% conversion of prior data as your default starting point.

Before getting to day zero when you will turn on the new system for full real use, it is imperative to request and establish a testing environment in addition to your live production environment. This allows you and your team to properly go through unit and integrated testing, working through any bugs and problems that arise, in a separate arena that will not disrupt the current clinical service work utilizing the live system.

System Configuration, Implementation Testing, and Validation

After you have established dual-environment arrangements, your team's next milestone is to arrange for your system to be configured with existing laboratory instrumentation as well as software interfaces with your EHR, clinical LIS, and outreach and reference sites. Once your system has been configured, the new setup can be tested and validated. The importance of this next order of business in establishing and completing a test plan cannot be understated—it can be the sole criterion on which your project is deemed a rousing success or an utter failure. Once a test plan is in place, complete with test procedures for each function that was approved and laid out in the system design deliberations as well as any interfaces that are modified or new, the ideal testing set should involve the system's new hardware and software configurations, working within anticipated security requirements and current clinical workflows.

Prior to go-live, validation of the system and its new functionality should take place wherein the gamut of anticipated potential clinical scenarios are put together and tested for both the ordering/input component of the transaction and the results/output transmittal side of the equation. Final, end-to-end integration testing incorporating order entry, result delivery, background financial processes, and associated interface crossing with test patients and their tracer specimens is needed to ensure that all the components of the system are present and verified to be in correct working order.

Training

Training involves a multitiered approached in which your team's project manager, the system manager(s), superuser(s), and designated trainer(s) are given initial instruction on the system, often at one of your selected vendor's training sites (with associated travel costs typically and presumptively built into your contract). This will allow for more extensive "train the trainer" preparation from the vendor directly and set your team leaders to become established to the point where they will be able to lead local training sessions for your end users. Be sure to inquire with the vendor about online modules or other remote training offerings that may obviate the time and financial burdens associated with training time. Whether distance training or not, be prepared to dedicate time slots for your laboratory's personnel to undergo this requisite commitment and have appropriate staffing coverage.

Go-Live

A few pragmatic items to mention before proceeding with your system's go-live revolve around communication and minimizing distractions. For the former, it is prudent to inform your client base (providers, outreach facilities, and the like) that you will be switching to a new system and that, although you do not anticipate any problems during the change, there may arise unforeseen hiccups during the transition. With regard to the latter, setting aside the go-live date for just your new system and avoiding any overlap with high-resource utilization periods, such as EHR installations, bringing on board new laboratory analyzers, or possible accreditation or inspection windows, is a preferred approach if such events are within your institution's control.

When the time has come to flip the switch on your new system, rest assured that you and your team's preparation and due diligence have set up for success. Granted there are postimplementation considerations surrounding issues of system maintenance or the inevitable workflow idiosyncrasy that is unique to your laboratory setting that the vendor's solution does not meet that will need to be addressed (and of course tested). But once you have reached this point, you can breathe easy—it will only be a few years before the refresh cycle comes full circle and you need to consider if and when to update your system again. Should you decide to do so, you will be better off having done it before and undoubtedly be better equipped with the lessons learned from the previous installation. We hope this article has helped you in modernizing one of the most important pieces of your laboratory's daily work.

REFERENCES

1. Anonymous. Available at: https://www.ftb.ca.gov/aboutFTB/Projects/ITSP/BPM_Glossary.pdf. Accessed June 23, 2014.
2. Sinard JH. Practical pathology informatics: demystifying informatics for the practicing anatomic pathologist. London: Springer-Verlag; 2006. p. 380.
3. Winsten D, Weiner H. Landing a new lis. Northfield: CAP Today; 2007. Available at: http://www.cap.org/apps//cap.portal?_nfpb=true%26cntvwrPtlt_actionOverride=%2Fportlets%2FcontentViewer%2Fshow%26_windowLabel=cntvwrPtlt%26cntvwrPtlt%7BactionForm.contentReference%7D=cap_today%2Ffeature_stories%2F0507NewLIS.html%26_state=maximized%26_pageLabel=cntvwr. Accessed July 15, 2014.
4. Sinard JH, Powell SZ, Karcher DS. Pathology training in informatics: evolving to meet a growing need. Arch Pathol Lab Med 2014;138(4):505–11.

Health Information Systems

S. Joseph Sirintrapun, MD[a],*, David R. Artz, MD[b]

KEYWORDS

- Laboratory information system • Health information systems
- Electronic medical record • Electronic health record
- Computerized provider order entry • Decision support

PART 1–A. HEALTH INFORMATION SYSTEMS—SETTINGS AND FUNCTIONS

Hospitals and health care organizations are complex systems comprising innumerable intricate operations and processes. Factoring advances in technology and medical knowledge, this complexity is further compounded. With such complexity, there is generation of immense amounts of information. Health information systems (HISs) are computing systems that capture, store, manage, or transmit this vast amount of information as it pertains to the health of individuals, clinical care, or the activities of health-related organizations. **Fig. 1** provides an overview of various HISs, which can be divided into 4 categories: (1) foundational systems, (2) financial systems, (3) departmental systems, and (4) electronic medical records (EMRs).

Foundational systems handle the managerial aspects for health care organizations and include the master patient index (MPI) and computing systems, which inform other HISs about admission, discharge, and transfer (ADT) activities. The transmitted message from an ADT system includes demographic information, such as name, date of birth, and gender. The MPI serves to index this information, like name, date of birth, gender, race, and social security number, ensuring that all registered patients are represented once without duplicate identities. The MPI also ensures consistent demographic information across all HISs within a health care organization.

This article originally appeared in Surgical Pathology Clinics, Volume 8, Issue 2, June 2015.
Disclosures: The authors have nothing to disclose.
[a] Department of Pathology, Memorial Sloan Kettering Cancer Center, 1275 York Avenue, New York, NY 10065, USA; [b] Memorial Sloan Kettering Cancer Center, 633 3rd Avenue, New York, NY 10017, USA
* Corresponding author.
E-mail address: sirintrs@mskcc.org

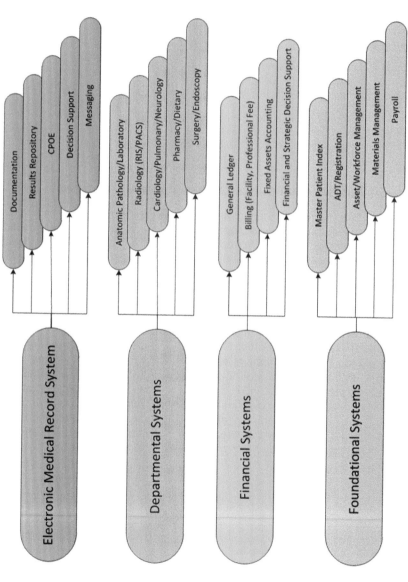

Fig. 1. Overview of HISs.

Financial systems handle the accounting aspects for a health-related organization and include billing systems, which handle hospital charges. The general ledger is another accounting system that serves as the backbone for financial and nonfinancial data. There are also financial systems that handle financial and strategic decision support (DS).

Departmental systems are computing systems that are specific to departmental needs and operations. The most visible system to surgical pathologists is the anatomic pathology laboratory information system (AP-LIS). The AP-LIS supports a vast array of operations and functionality for the anatomic pathology laboratory. As a counterpart, the clinical laboratory has the clinical laboratory information system, which frequently is not interoperable with the AP-LIS. Radiology has the radiology information system (RIS), which deals with patient lists, patient tracking, orders, workflows, and results entry with reporting. Serving in conjunction with the RIS in radiology is the picture archiving and communication system, which manages the large repository of radiologic images. Cardiology also has its own version, separate from that in radiology, which handles cardiology images, such as echocardiograms and cardiac catheterization procedures. There are departmental systems for departments that perform specialized testing (ie, ECGs in cardiology, pulmonary function tests for pulmonology, and electromyograms for neurology). Some institutions may bring various imaging modalities together in a separate system, called a vendor neutral archive. Departmental systems exist for pharmacy and dietary departments to streamline workflows by handling medication and dietary orders, coordination administration, and distribution.

Clinical laboratories and financial management departments were the first to adopt HISs. Other types of HISs sprouted to reflect the operational and functional needs of their respective departments. As a consequence of this subspecialization, however, HISs developed independently in silos and with their own individual database infrastructure. This occurred with the AP-LIS and the clinical laboratory information system, and the consequence was a lack of interoperable HISs that do not interface or interact with each other seamlessly. There are other reasons for this lack of interoperability, such as lack of standardization for interoperability. Vendors of departmental HISs had incentive to create dependency of health care organizations and not come together to create interoperable standards with other competing vendors. This ethos continued until recently where forces advocating for interoperability had become strong enough to influence policy.

The realization for the breakdown of silos and having a more interoperable HISs was not a recent idea, but began as early as 1991. Then, the Institute of Medicine (IOM) set forth a vision and issued a strong call for nationwide implementation of computer-based patient records.[1] The IOM acknowledged that physician groups, hospitals, and other health care organizations operated as silos, often providing care without the benefit of complete information about a patient's condition, medical history, services provided in other settings, or medications prescribed by other clinicians.[2] The IOM called for interoperability through automation and linking of information on services provided to patients in ambulatory and institutional settings (eg, encounters, procedures, and ancillary tests). This interoperability would in turn provide a rich source of information for quality measurement and improvement purposes to enable quality integrated clinical care.[2]

Because of reports like those issued by the IOM, there has been recent widespread adoption of EMRs. Most importantly, federal incentive programs have targeted EMRs to redesign the health care system to create quality integrated clinical care. The EMR is discussed later.

Key Points

- There are 4 categories of HISs
  - Foundational systems
  - Financial systems
  - Departmental systems
  - EMR

- Pressure for HIS interoperability is not new, but only recently with aid of federal incentive programs, has there been push for redesign of the health care system to create quality integrated clinical care.

- This has led to widespread adoption of EMRs.

PART 1–B. HEALTH INFORMATION SYSTEMS—ARCHETYPAL ARCHITECTURES

Interoperability by HISs occurs by 2 archetypal architectures: (1) integrated systems and (2) interfaced systems. Integrated systems are those in which data are housed in the same database and used by various HISs (ie, departmental, financial, and foundational). Interfaced systems are those where HISs are separate applications and data are housed in their own databases. Data are communicated between each separate system through an interface engine usually using a Health Level Seven International 7 (HL7) protocol. Most of the U.S. healthcare organizations are on some iteration of Version 2 for HL7; otherwise specified as HL7 Version 2.x (V2). The significance of HL7 Version 2.x (V2) will be addressed later. Valid arguments exist for both archetypal architectures in terms of advantages and disadvantages.

With integrated systems, information flow is theoretically more seamless because of the foundation of one database. Imagine an integrated system for anatomic pathology, clinical laboratory, and molecular pathology in reporting a hypothetical bone marrow core specimen. Currently such an optimized integrated system does not exist. Under an optimized integrated system however, a pathology report on a bone marrow core can be generated from the AP-LIS with seamless incorporation of a complete blood count (CBC) and/or aspirate result from the clinical laboratory information system. Once the ancillary molecular test results return, an addendum can be tagged into the report, all transactions happening hypothetically under one application without need for different logins, copy-paste actions, or correcting formatting issues.

There is a general sense, however, that integrated systems are not optimized for operational and functional needs of departments. Large vendors are better positioned to create integrated systems but by their size are believed less focused or receptive to the operational and functional needs of each individual department. Large vendors also are thought less nimble to handle nuanced changes that enhance applications. Moreover, because these integrated systems are built on one database, small changes in one application can have unforeseen downstream consequences to the other integrated applications. Along the same lines, integrated systems are more vulnerable to disruption. Corruptions to the database, downtimes, or upgrades affect all applications because they are not able to function independently. The theoretic simplification that occurs because disparate systems run on the same database is a selling point of integrated systems.

With interfaced systems, departments can keep their own departmental HIS, which often addresses the operational and functional needs of respective department more optimally. The term, *best of breed*, derives from the description of such departmental systems. Most of the nuances and customizations demanded by departments may be handled more effectively with a best of breed system. Best of breed systems usually stem from smaller more nimble vendors with incentives for self-preservation to make the most optimized system in their domain. Often such vendors are more receptive and better able to handle changes to their products.

Interfaced systems are heavily dependent on well-implemented communication and routing. This is the reason why more testing is required under such archetypal architecture. In practice, even under the best interfaced system, interoperability is never really fully achieved. With the same scenario under an interfaced system, having an integrated report for the same bone marrow core becomes more difficult. A pathology report on a bone marrow core is generated from an AP-LIS, but there is no seamless incorporation of CBC and/or aspirate result from the clinical laboratory information system. Tagging a molecular addendum poses a similar challenge. The sign-out process mandates separate logins and, once results are obtained, mechanisms for transferring the results to the AP-LIS are usually copy-paste. Without seamless automation for results transfer, errors can occur. The overall sign-out process becomes disruptive because of the different logins, copy-paste actions, and correcting of formatting issues.

In practice, most organizational clinical computing systems are combinations of integrated and interfaced systems, with varying degrees of each. In an ideal world, an integrated system should be optimized for the operational and functional needs of departments. Likewise, an interfaced system should have the seamless modes of interfacing between various applications.

Key Points

- Two archetypal architectures
  - Integrated systems
    - Advantages: one database, more interoperabilty
    - Disadvantages: arguably less customized functionality, more vulnerability of disruption due to interdependency, changes/upgrades more difficult due to interdependency (entire enterprise affected)
  - Interfaced systems
    - Advantages: arguably more customized functionality, less vulnerability to disruptions, changes/upgrades can be staggered and are more manageable (only portions of the enterprise affected)
    - Disadvantages: multiple databases, less interoperability, interface engine dependent

---

PART 2. ELECTRONIC MEDICAL RECORD SYSTEMS AS A FOUNDATIONAL TOOL

The Committee on Quality of Health Care in America in 2001 called for health care organizations to aim for health care that is safe, effective, timely, efficient, equitable, and patient centered. This would require greater access to shared information, expanding communication channels, and overcoming sociotechnical challenges. This also spelled a key role for information technology. Only through support from carefully and consciously designed information systems would health care be enabled to meet these aims.[2] The solution was the EMR, which acts as a foundational tool by helping users better integrate, distribute, organize, interpret, and react to health information and knowledge. **Table 1** lists the advantages and disadvantages of the EMR.

There will be much discussion of the value added by EMRs; however, a few of the disadvantages should be highlighted. EMRs can be expensive. There often seems to

Table 1
Advantages and disadvantages of the electronic medical record

Advantages	Disadvantages

• Integrative virtual work environment
• Accessibility and availability
  ○ Portable
  ○ Multiple user view
• Messaging and alerts
• Patient care safety
  ○ Legibility
  ○ Audit trails
• Error reduction
  ○ Computerized order entry
  ○ Computerized Decision Support
• Information capture and management
  ○ Quality improvement
  ○ Research
	• Costly
	• Training
	• User resistance
	• Workflow disruption (ie, electronic note entry and documentation)
	• Inadequate results display
	• Technical issues (ie, network, interface)

be a level of technical familiarity as prerequisite in using EMRs. There are costs in training because EMRs are not necessarily designed to be intuitive for less computer savvy individuals. Workflow disruptions are also notable, particularly with electronic notes, which have had many reported downsides. Data entry for documentation via clicking, typing, and scrolling may take some users longer than scribbling on paper.[3]

The advantages of an EMR in terms of its functionalities seem to override the obstacles. A well-designed and functioning EMR further enables users to utilize this health information and knowledge to influence policy and decision-making, action, individual and public health outcomes, and research. The functionalities of the EMR are listed in **Box 1** and discussed in sequence.[4]

ADMINISTRATIVE PROCESSES

Depending on the health care organization, foundational and financial systems can occur as separate HISs interfaced with the EMR. With such interface types of architecture, extensive testing is required to ensure that the care that occurred along with the documentation noted in the EMR coincides and matches correctly with the billing codes and list of patients and providers in the foundational and financial systems.

Box 1
Functionalities for the electronic medical record

• Administrative processes

• Centralization of health information and knowledge

• Results management

• Messaging (electronic communication and connectivity)

• Computerized Provider Order Entry

• Decision Support

• Patient support

• Data capture, reporting, and population health management

EMRs have evolved to incorporate the functionalities of foundational and financial systems in an integrated manner. This integration of foundational and financial HISs to manage documentation for regulatory, compliance, quality assurance, and billing ends up being the back end of modern EMRs.[5]

CENTRALIZATION OF HEALTH INFORMATION AND KNOWLEDGE

The front end of the EMR is the most visible system to clinicians and patients. It is this front end that is ubiquitous in numerous clinical settings (listed in **Table 2**).

The EMR serves as an integrative work environment, centralizing health information for display and presentation. Much like the paper chart, health information is acquired, collected, collated, and stored from other information systems like the AP-LIS. But beyond a paper chart, the EMR is accessible, portable, and available—factors that have been the source of physician satisfaction with such an information system. The EMR has enhanced the practice of surgical pathology. EMRs overcome the issues of accessibility and portability of paper charts, such as physical filing and retrieving of information and misplacement. No longer is there a need to request a paper chart or call or e-mail for clinical correlation. Health information is available during all 24 hours and multiple users can access a single patient record on demand, which is a difficult task with a paper chart.

RESULTS MANAGEMENT

For surgical pathology, results management translates into how surgical pathology reports are presented in the EMR. Surgical pathology reports are reconstructed visually in the EMR through HL7 Version 2.x (V2) messaging and rendered in unformatted text. This translation results in style and formatting loss in the rendered EMR report. EMR reports are not able to handle bold, italics, colors, tables, figures, or pictures. The HL7 Version 2.x (V2) messaging standard rendering reports in an EMR works best for laboratory reports, which are shorter and less textual than surgical pathology reports. The HL7 Version 2.x (V2) messaging standard was not intended to display surgical pathology reports in an intuitive layout. Surgical pathology reports are considerably longer; consider tumor resections with long synoptic checklists. The beautiful reports generated by genitourinary and molecular diagnostic laboratories are not readily reconstructed in the same manner in institutional EMRs. Pathologists, who aligned their data through an aligned column format in Microsoft Word, are often surprised that the information displayed in the EMR does not maintain alignments well. An even more dangerous example is with certain symbols like " ~ ", where the words

Table 2	
Electronic medical record settings	
• Ambulatory clinic	• Inpatient
• Outpatient surgical center	○ Acute care
• Emergency room	○ Psychiatry
• Operating room	○ Rehabilitation service
• Skilled nursing facility	○ ICU
• Long-term acute care facility	▪ Trauma/surgical
• Home	▪ Pulmonology
	▪ Cardiology
	▪ Neurology/neurosurgery
	▪ Neonatal

that follow the symbol can be deleted. Thus statements like " ~ no carcinoma identi-fied" become "carcinoma identified." Pathologists should be aware of the representa-tion of their reports in the EMR and not just from the AP-LIS. In addition it is the responsibility under Clinical Laboratory Improvement Amendments (CLIA) of a labora-tory to know how the results are displayed in the EMR and, if there are multiple insti-tutional EMRs, that results are consistent. Pathologists should be aware of where the results of their generated reports are mapped in the EMR and if there are possibilities for hidden results under any permutation.[5]

Having surgical pathology reports that are human readable and easier to compre-hend rapidly proves increasingly difficult with the onset of advanced molecular testing with next-generation sequencing (NGS). NGS is inherently complicated and intuitive layouts presumably require figures, graphs, tables, charts, and so forth, in contrast to unstructured paragraphs of text. Even worse, NGS, unlike the cancer checklists for reporting, has no established guidelines for reporting NGS information. To enhance reporting capabilities in the EMR, some institutions have implemented a PDF interface to overcome the limitations of HL7 Version 2.x (V2) reconstructed reports. The report in PDF format is good for complex reporting because it enables intuitive layouts with ca-pabilities of including bold and colors and the ability to recreate figures, graphs, tables, charts, and so forth. Not only does this avert misinterpretation through formatting and transmission errors but also it becomes a form of passive clinical decision support (discussed later).

Implementing a PDF interface from an AP-LIS requires partnerships from informa-tion technology teams from other HISs within the institution, notably the interface en-gine and the EMR. Many EMRs do not have the functionality to display PDFs or do not have the functionality readily available. Moreover, institutions with data warehouses might resist the idea because PDFs only display and render information that is not easily data mineable. To circumvent such concerns, processes should be ensured to all parties that data streams are maintained if current information mining processes are in place. **Fig. 2** is one example of an institution's information workflow, which has enabled PDF functionality. When the Microsoft Word Document is created from the sign-out in the AP-LIS, this triggers creation of a PDF version that sits on an accessible institutional server. The HL7 Version 2.x (V2) message that is created after the sign-out of the report then contains a pointer field, which triggers the EMR to retrieve the PDF document for display into the EMR. The institutional data warehouse, in this example, captures information through parsing the HL7 Version 2.x (V2) message and thus the feeder data stream is maintained. As value added for clinical care, a polished PDF report is rendered for display in the EMR.

The PDF interface represents the first stage in enhanced reporting and arguably passive decision support. It can act as the enhanced reporting solution within the con-fines of HL7 Version 2.x (V2). The next stage in reporting may come through the concept of clinical document architecture (CDA). The current iterations of HL7 Version 2.x (V2) do not encompass CDA. Rather CDA is a component of HL7 Version 3 (V3) which is the next generation of HL7 messaging. CDA was intended for transmission standards to take into account the structural components of clinical documents, in particular the clinical visit note, which is highly textual. Clinical visit notes are not just accumulated lines of text but also documents with structural components, such as the physical examination, review of systems, and assessment and plan section. Surgical pathology reports, also highly textual, can be considered analogous to clinical visit notes with structural components like the final diagnosis section, gross descrip-tion section, addendum section, and so forth. CDA provides organizational context for how reports are structured and positioned and standardizes the appearance of

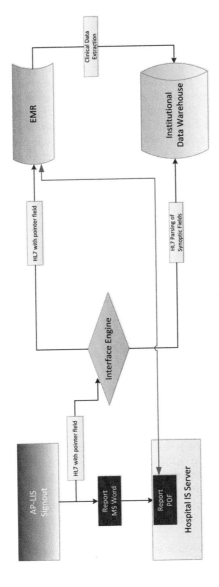

Fig. 2. Information flow for an Institution which enabled PDF functionality.

documents in the EMR.[6] The advantage over a PDF interface is that with CDA capability, the data stream or report rendered EMR becomes more structured and more amenable to processing and data mining unlike the unstructured PDF. Fortunately, CDA functionality is likely to appear in all US commercial EMRs because this functionality is included in the requirements for meaningful use under the United States HITECH Act. Whether this implementation of CDA occurs through adoption of HL7 Version 3 (V3) remains unclear however due mainly to the hesitancy of EMR vendors to adopt towards HL7 Version 3 (V3) standards.

The reasons for EMR vendors not adopting HL7 Version 3 (V3) standards are multifactorial. Because EMR vendors of today are large and widely implemented, the competition incentive to evolve toward better messaging standards is absent. Such vendor systems also create a higher reliance and interdependency. Because all components of such vendor systems are interdependent, developments and improvements have unintended consequences throughout the system, making even incremental developments harder to implement. In short, systems become too big to improve and disruptive or even revolutionary changes are even harder to incorporate. There are also prohibitive costs in terms of infrastructure changes to the EMR for adoption of an HL7 Version 3 (V3) standard. HL7 Version 3 (V3) is not backwards compatible with HL7 Version 2.x (V2). This was by design because the intent of HL7 Version 3 (V3) was to be completely revolutionary and not to be hamstrung by the legacy constraints of HL7 Version 2.x (V2). Further compounding is the fact that HL7 Version 3 (V3) is highly complex and experience for implementation is still immature. In other words, there are growing pains with adopting something new like the HL7 Version 3 (V3), pains that EMR vendors are reluctant to take on unless further pressured. Because of the difficulties with adoption of HL7 Version 3 (V3) by EMR vendors, the implementation of CDA may occur through modalities like Fast Healthcare Interoperability Resources (FHIR). The discussion of FHIR is beyond the scope of this article, however a simplified view of FHIR is of a hybrid messaging solution. FHIR can act as a standalone messaging standard and encompass many of the beneficial functionalities of HL7 Version 3 (V3), like CDA. The advantage over HL7 Version 3 (V3) is that FHIR can be used in partnership with current HL7 Version 2.x (V2) standards.

Surgical pathology reports are in need of more dynamic capabilities for managing updates. Updates on reports often come in the form of addendums. The pathology specimen is signed out as the initial report, and then ancillary testing is performed with results usually tagged at the end of the initial report. This is sufficient for a 1-time study, like an immunohistochemical predictive/prognostic panel performed on, for example, a breast specimen. But if there are multiple tests performed on multiple parts of a specimen, tagging addendums to the end of a report makes the report layout less intuitive. NGS poses this dilemma because NGS can be run on multiple tumor sites listed as different parts within a specimen. Ideally, tagging an addendum to its associated part is the most intuitive layout; however, this requires parts to be separated as components of the final diagnosis section, which is a functionality that most AP-LIS vendors lack.

With genomic reporting, AP-LISs are simply not ready because there are too many unresolved issues. Information, such as the performance characteristics of an assay or whether an assay is single analyte versus multiparametric, is difficult to convey. There are questions in reporting mutations or in negative results and regarding whether sequence information, such as location, sequencing depth, sequencing quality, and regions interrogated, should be stored. Current communication interfacing standards with HL7 Version 2.x (V2) do not support data formatting and metadata for genomic information, such that only dumbed-down genomic results are reportable.

For now, the PDF interface represents the best mechanism to perform enhanced pathology reporting with CDA to occur sometime in the future. This somewhat over-comes the current limitations that current communication interfacing standards have imposed with conveying information in a graphical or interactive manner. Perhaps the optimal solution to enhanced reporting will come from an application pro-gram interface (API), which utilizes hyperlinks in an HTML Web-based manner for dis-tribution of information to and from an EMR. The advantage is that information and reports can be updated dynamically, thus creating truly interactive reports. There also will be the ability to deliver report metadata, limitations for interpretation, and level of evidence for interpretation through background and references on demand.

Key Points

- Surgical pathology reports are reconstructed visually in an EMR through HL7 Version 2.x (V2) messaging and rendered in unformatted text.

- HL7 Version 2.x (V2) messaging standard was not intended to display surgical pathology reports in an intuitive layout.

- Responsibility under CLIA resides with the laboratory to know how the results are displayed in the EMR and, if there are multiple institutional EMRs, that results are consistent.

- HL7 Version 2.x (V2) messaging proves more inadequate for NGS reporting with possible solutions including a PDF interface, further development of CDA, or evolution toward a more interactive HTML-based API.

- Updates of reports, as with ancillary testing with NGS, are future issues because tagging addenda to the ends of reports is not ideal

---

MESSAGING (ELECTRONIC COMMUNICATION AND CONNECTIVITY)

It is no longer sufficient to just render a pathology report in an EMR and assume that all of the clinical team is aware and receiving the information adequately, particularly when there are updates on reports. Clinical care, now that it is more integrated, man-dates various clinical teams and personnel receiving updated information about mul-tiple patients. Managing when, who, and where the reports with any updates are routed is paramount. This poses a difficult challenge in how EMRs handle transmitted information of reports with updates, notably addenda.

Often the associated submitting provider for a pathology specimen is not the person the updated information in the addenda is intended for. Some EMRs lack functionality to alert the appropriate provider for such updates. If a breast lumpectomy specimen is signed out, the submitting surgeon is fine with knowing the final pathology with resec-tion margin status. If NGS is requested by an oncologist on the same specimen, how-ever, and then there is a handover in care to another oncologist provider, routing the results of an NGS addenda to the new oncology provider is considerably difficult. Catastrophic errors can occur if results are not relayed appropriately, with certain crucial members of a clinical team unaware of actionable test results.

EMRs are getting better with managing changing providers and distribution of infor-mation, but alerting mechanisms via the EMR for updated pathology reports is still a work in progress. Some EMRs are able to do group providers involved in care such that alerts for results go to the entire group to enhance electronic communication with the clinical team. Idealized EMRs would track chain of custody of care, but alter-native mechanisms include messaging capabilities for providers, such as an inbox, or-ders to approve, results to acknowledge, and forwarding mechanisms, such as faxes, printing, and transmission to other systems. Unfortunately some EMRs in use today lack such robust forwarding capabilities, and, even if present, mechanisms are not well established to determine the appropriate provider to forward results to.

Key Points

- It is insufficient to just render a pathology report in the EMR without knowing how the results are received adequately.
- Managing when, who, and where the reports, with any updates, are routed is paramount.
- Results routing is a future challenge for how EMRs handle transmitted information of reports with updates, notably addenda.
- Idealized EMRs would track chain of custody of care, but alternative mechanisms include messaging capabilities for providers, such as an inbox, orders to approve, results to acknowledge, and forwarding mechanisms, such as faxes, printing, and transmission to other systems.

COMPUTERIZED PROVIDER ORDER ENTRY

Computerized provider order entry (CPOE) is a process that allows an ordering provider to use a computer to directly enter medications, procedures, orders, consultations, and tests, notably radiology and laboratory. Orders are entered in the EMR, and the system then transmits this order over a network via HL7.

From a quality and safety perspective, CPOE has shown a reduction in medical errors. In a study by Bates and colleagues,[7] medical ordering errors were cut by more than half. CPOE reduces errors through (1) eliminating misinterpretation through illegible handwriting or transcription; (2) readily identifying the ordering provider; (3) minimizing inappropriate, unnecessary, or redundant tests; and (4) ensuring that sufficient information is included with orders and improves compliance with medical staff policies. **Fig. 3** shows an example of a CPOE menu for ordering an NGS panel on a surgical pathology tumor specimen. In addition to eliminating misinterpretation through illegible handwriting on paper requisitions, the order provider is readily identifiable, and the system does not allow for duplicate orders if an order is already placed. In addition, the order cannot be processed until sufficient information is placed into certain menu items.

The AP-LISs of today unfortunately lack interface capability for CPOE with EMRs. Moreover, hospital systems are not designed or have not developed workflow to handle the components of a well-implemented CPOE for surgical pathology, such as bar code printing, scanning, and distribution at point of tissue acquisition. Instead of an electronic order, workflows of today usually begin with specimen and paper requisition delivered at an accessioning point, which eventually ends with reports displayed in an EMR. This describes an unclosed loop because the pathology report does not end up at the beginning with an electronic order through CPOE in the EMR. As a consequence, data prior to the point of accession (preanalytical variables) are not captured or evaluated. **Fig. 4** shows an idealized CPOE interface with an AP-LIS, which has created a closed loop with the report, ending back at the beginning with an order entered in CPOE. By closing the loop, CPOE enables for a transition to a paperless workflow with bar codes printed at the point of tissue acquisition for transport to pathology accessioning points. CPOE for surgical pathology specimens opens the door for application of business analytics, where preanalytical data are captured such time as from electronic order to specimen receipt in the laboratory and tracking data when bar codes are scanned from locations prior to the pathology accessioning point.

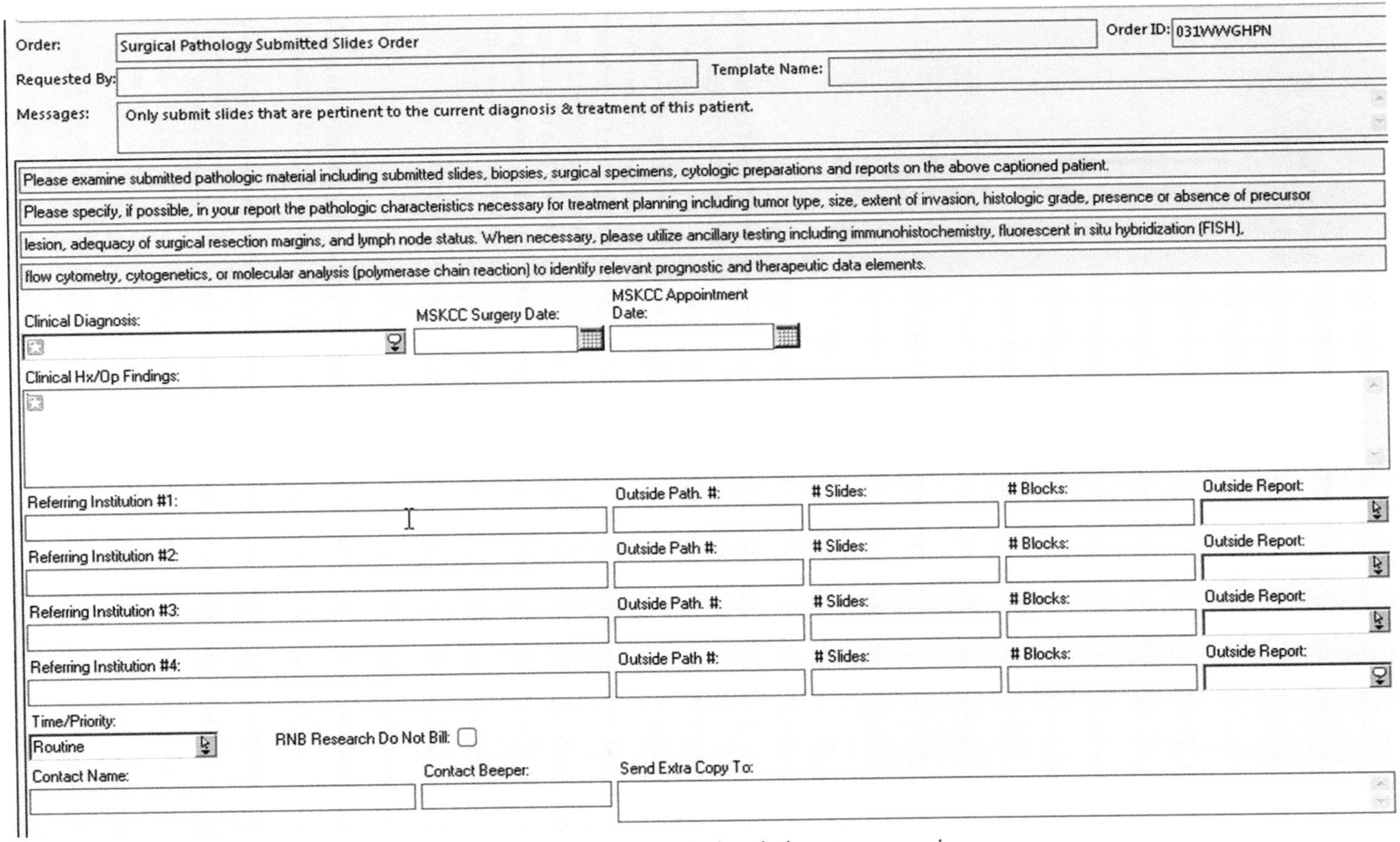

Order: | Surgical Pathology Submitted Slides Order | Order ID: | 03YWVGHPN

Requested By:

Template Name:

Messages: | Only submit slides that are pertinent to the current diagnosis & treatment of this patient.

Please examine submitted pathologic material including submitted slides, biopsies, surgical specimens, cytologic preparations and reports on the above captioned patient.

Please specify, if possible, in your report the pathologic characteristics necessary for treatment planning including tumor type, size, extent of invasion, histologic grade, presence or absence of precursor lesion, adequacy of surgical resection margins, and lymph node status. When necessary, please utilize ancillary testing including immunohistochemistry, fluorescent in situ hybridization (FISH), flow cytometry, cytogenetics, or molecular analysis (polymerase chain reaction) to identify relevant prognostic and therapeutic data elements.

Clinical Diagnosis:

MSKCC Surgery Date: | MSKCC Appointment Date:

Clinical Hx/Op Findings:

Referring Institution #1: | Outside Path. #: | Outside Path #: | # Slides: | # Blocks: | Outside Report:

Referring Institution #2: | Outside Path #: | # Slides: | # Blocks: | Outside Report:

Referring Institution #3: | Outside Path. #: | # Slides: | # Blocks: | Outside Report:

Referring Institution #4: | Outside Path #: | # Slides: | # Blocks: | Outside Report:

Time/Priority: | Routine

RNB Research Do Not Bill

Contact Name: | Contact Beeper: | Send Extra Copy To:

Fig. 3. Screenshot of a CPOE menu for ordering an NGS panel on a surgical pathology tumor specimen.

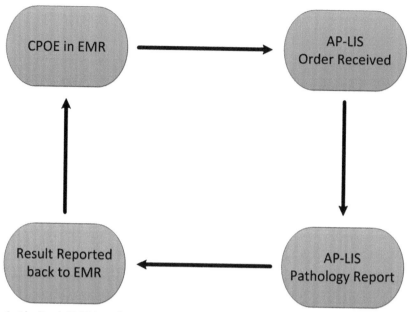

Fig. 4. Idealized CPOE interface with an AP-LIS.

A useful tool in CPOE is the order set. Order sets involve grouping of orders with intent to standardize and expedite the ordering process for a common clinical scenario. The rationale for order sets is provided in **Box 2**.[8]

Fig. 5 shows an order set on an NGS panel, which requires both matched tumor on a surgical pathology specimen and a normal blood sample. The largest confounding variable is that tumor and the matched normal blood sample are obtained at different times and locations. Without CPOE, coordinating whether a paper requisition for tumor was filled appropriately along with a normal blood sample, which has its own paper requisition, becomes a logistical nightmare. This menu centralizes the ordering of such a panel while reducing the probability of a provider mistakenly reordering the test. It also enables compliance with the institutional practice standard that both matched tumor and normal samples be obtained for the test to proceed.

DECISION SUPPORT

Decision support (DS) enables providers with knowledge and patient-specific information. Idealized DS is intelligently filtered and presented in a timely fashion. DS

Box 2
Rationale for order sets

- Reduce time required to enter orders
- Reduce errors and increase accuracy during order entry
- Increase completeness of orders
- Built-in DS and evidence-driven care
- Reduce variability in the care process and enhance compliance with best practices

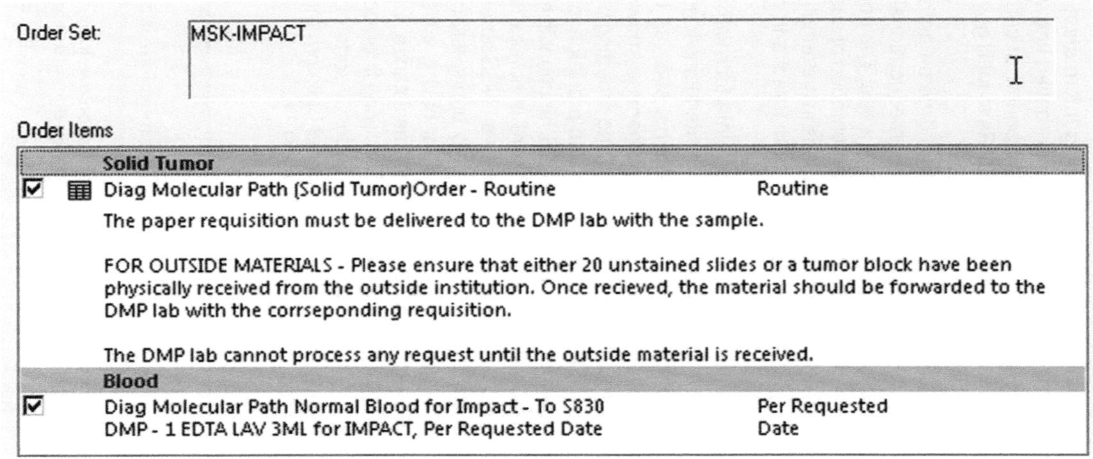

Order Set: MSK-IMPACT

Order Items

Solid Tumor

▶ ▦ Diag Molecular Path [Solid Tumor]Order - Routine   Routine

The paper requisition must be delivered to the DMP lab with the sample.

FOR OUTSIDE MATERIALS - Please ensure that either 20 unstained slides or a tumor block have been physically received from the outside institution. Once recieved, the material should be forwarded to the DMP lab with the corrseponding requisition.

The DMP lab cannot process any request until the outside material is received.

Blood

▶ Diag Molecular Path Normal Blood for Impact - To S830   Per Requested
DMP - 1 EDTA LAV 3ML for IMPACT, Per Requested Date   Date

Fig. 5. Screenshot of a NGS order set at MSKCC.

encompasses a variety of tools to enhance decision making, including computerized alerts and reminders to providers, clinical guidelines, condition-specific order sets, documentation templates, diagnostic support, and contextually relevant reference information.[9] As discussed previously with reporting of NGS results, a focused PDF report and summary can be a passive version of DS. Many institutions already have implemented a PDF interface as a component of their clinical reporting of NGS to integrate back in EMRs.[10]

DS is becoming necessary to address the growing information overload clinicians face and to provide a platform for integrating evidence-based knowledge into care delivery. A majority of DS applications operate as components of comprehensive EMRs. DS is also becoming the reason for implementing EMRs to fulfill government mandates for meaningful use.

DS is often coupled with CPOE, where electronic orders can be linked to clinical guidelines, contextually relevant reference information educational content, and rules engines to check orders (duplicates) and to generate alerts. The condition-specific order set seen in **Fig. 5** is also a form of DS. The implementation of such menus improves physician ordering patterns by locking down variations in ordering habits. In **Fig. 5**, order for an NGS panel cannot be processed unless both tumor and normal samples are checked and requested.

DS is not without its hurdles. Ideally, DS applications interface with the AP-LIS; however, most AP-LIS vendors have not yet developed such interfacing functionality. DS also, if poorly designed, creates inefficiency with interruptions, such as too many pop-ups, warnings, hurdles, and alerts to initiating an order, otherwise known as "alert fatigue." DS is seen as a necessary component of NGS testing and reporting because DS systems can use panomic data to guide treatment selection and precision medicine.[11] Currently there are several necessary integrated CPOE and DS functionalities that are not supported by current EMRs to enable NGS testing. There is no seamless mechanism to have records for consent and counseling conveyed to an NGS laboratory. For germline genetic testing, there is no mechanism to ensure no unnecessary expensive repeat testing, such as referring to a preexisting test result or having a lifetime duplicate test check rule. Complex tests, such as NGS, do require assistance. Clinicians should not be held to a level of sophistication of knowing when ordering fluorescence in situ hybridization (FISH), karyotyping, or NGS is appropriate under all sorts of scenarios. Another large hurdle is the lack of standards to enable powerful bioinformatics tools like variant databases to interface with DS applications in the EMR.[10]

Key Points

- DS enables providers with knowledge and patient-specific information and ideally DS is intelligently filtered and timely presented.

- DS is becoming necessary to address the growing information overload clinicians face and to provide a platform for integrating evidence-based knowledge into care delivery.

- Clinicians should not be held to a level of sophistication of knowing when ordering FISH, karyotyping, or NGS is appropriate under all sorts of scenarios.

- DS hurdles
  - DS applications do not interface with the AP-LIS.
  - Several necessary integrated CPOE and DS functionalities are not supported by current EMRs to enable NGS testing.
  - There is a lack of standards to enable powerful bioinformatics tools like variant databases to interface with DS applications in the EMR.

PATIENT SUPPORT

In discussing patient support, the concept of a patient portal is introduced. A patient portal is a secure online Web site that gives patients convenient 24-hour access to personal health information from anywhere with an Internet connection. EMRs of today are implementing patient portals to enhance patient-provider communication, empower patients, support care between visits, and, most importantly, improve patient outcomes. Patient portals are seen as a solution to meet the expectations of stage 1 of meaningful use in engaging patients in their own health care.[12] Many patient portals display laboratory results, but surgical pathology reports raise another set of issues.

From the surgical pathologist perspective, when and how pathology reports are displayed in a patient portal become issues. If a patient has a resection for a tumor, what is the appropriate time for the report to be displayed in the portal? If the report is displayed too soon, the patient may not see the provider in time for a discussion about issues about prognosis. How the report is displayed is also important. Would a patient be able to interpret a pathology report written for clinicians, or will that lead to more questions fielded by clinicians or potentially even pathologists.

As implementation of patient portals becomes more widespread, should a more patient-focused report with appropriate language and terminology be done and would this create more issues than it resolves because it can potentially lead to an interpretative discrepancy between the official pathology report and the patient-focused one? An optimized solution or model has has yet to be introduced.

Key Points

- Patient portals are seen as a solution to meet the expectations of stage 1 of meaningful use in engaging patients in their own health care.
- There are many issues that arise and are unresolved with the advent of patient portals.
- Pathologists should be active in the management of results in patient portals.

DATA CAPTURE, REPORTING, AND POPULATION HEALTH MANAGEMENT

Early EMRs could be thought of as an enhanced electronic version of the paper chart because they are able to provide secure, real-time, current, interactive, and portable information on an individual. Because of this focus on the individual, the EMR is considered patient centric because it operates within 1 health care organization and is more focused on episodes/encounters and immediate health care, like clinical information collected from a provider's office.[5]

Another term that is used interchangeably, although mistakenly, is electronic health record (EHR). EMRs and EHRs have similar functionality because they both work as enhanced electronic versions of paper charts. EHRs are more longitudinal, encompassing the entirety of a patient's episodes/encounters and across health care organizations. Unlike EMRs, EHRs can encompass more than just the one health care organization that originally collected and compiled the information. They are built to share information with other health care providers, such as laboratories and specialists, so they contain information from all the clinicians involved in the patient's care. In theory, the EHR enables the ability to easily share medical information among stakeholders and to have a patient's information follow that person through the various modalities of care engaged by that individual. Information can move with the patient—to a specialist, a hospital, a nursing home, the next state, or even across the country. This allows for comparison of various records of an individual and allows for extraction of data from records across different individuals. This mobility of information enables EHRs to go beyond the health and immediate patient-centric health care, toward the goal of bettering population health. The heart of a well-implemented HER is sophisticated data capture, which is amenable to computer processing.[13]

An immense wealth of data is contained in the databases of EMRs/EHRs; consider clinical notes and reports from laboratory, pathology, and radiology. Countless other types of data elements are captured by the EMR/EHR, such as clinic visit dates, blood pressure readings, and vaccinations. Such data can be tracked over time and used to check on how patients are doing and to identify which patients due for screenings or checkups. Through this monitoring of captured data, EMRs/EHRs, in concept, improve overall quality of care within the health organization. With even more advanced queries and monitoring of EMR/EHR database and the mobility of the extracted data from different records, information can be used for audits, research, outcomes assessment, research, and surveillance. The ability to use this information in more meaningful ways to elucidate insight and knowledge is a key goal of EHRs.

With this promise for better overall health care for individuals and population health, there are obstacles that require solutions before the full potential of EHRs is achieved in the setting of improving health care of individuals and of population health. EMRs, despite containing immense wealth in data, have most of the data captured unstructured and not easily amenable to computer processing. This is usually not an issue with data elements, like clinical visit dates, blood pressures, and laboratory data, which are often short, numeric, and less textual. For data elements contained in textual documents, such as clinical notes and pathology reports, however, the accumulated lines of text in some EMRs provide little structure or context to create parsing algorithms to mine and extract the data. An example is capturing data from a family history section of a clinical note for familial correlations of disease processes. The family history is sometimes reported as accumulated lines of text that offer no structure or context to a computer. Graphical representation with family trees hypothetically is a better mechanism for data capture; however, this functionality is far from universal.

The narrative text-based format of sections like the family history may change in the future with meaningful use by mandating that EMRs capture data better through more structured mechanisms. CDA, as discussed previously, may be a step forward and holds promise for such structured capture. For now, however, templates can lock down the structure of certain data elements of a document. Synoptic reporting of cancer specimens has been widely implemented and easily utilized and applied. Because of the consistency and structure of the information, these synoptic cancer templates have structured lines of text in a manner amenable to computer processing. Templates for many EMR clinic notes have received mixed reactions, with the downside a limitation on flexibility in applying the template to nuanced situations. This basically forces documentation into frameworks without the ability to tailor for clinical exceptions.

Referring to **Fig. 2**, an institution that possesses a data warehouse has created mechanisms for clinical data extraction from the EMR database to provide clinical correlations while also enabling parsing algorithms to capture data from synoptic templates in cancer pathology reports from the transmitted HL7 Version 2.x (V2) message. In this way, the institution is able to create a streamlined automated information flow, which coordinates the association between clinical data, such as clinical trials and treatment, with the cancer reporting elements into the institutional data warehouse.

As mechanisms improve for capturing data, EHRs will also continue to evolve better transmission mechanisms to public health databases focused on reportable diseases to better population health. This reporting to public health agencies for more global surveillance of disease is also mandated under meaningful use. Consider the reporting of infectious diseases for outbreak surveillance as well as tumor cases for cancer registries. Such tasks were difficult in the days of paper records, but now, using captured data elements in EHRs, transferring directly to cloud-based public health data centers with their own information systems is more seamless.

Key Points

- Information sharing is the ultimate key goal of EHRs with the hope of improving the quality of health in the population.

- Mobility of the extracted data from different records can enable information to be used for audits, research, outcomes assessment, research, and surveillance.

- Extracted and shared information can be evaluated toward more meaningful ways to elucidate insight and knowledge.

- Cancer synoptic reporting helps enable better and more automated data sharing for public databases, such as cancer registries.

SUMMARY

Pathologists have become gatekeepers of tissue and information. Pathologists must acknowledge their role in quality integrated clinical care and engage information system teams outside of the departmental AP-LIS. EMRs/EHRs are developing functionalities for which pathologists should be stakeholders to provide valuable pathology domain knowledge. This requires moving out of the traditional siloed mind-set and collaborating with clinical colleagues, administrative teams, and vendors as part of institutional information system teams to coordinate efficient flows for information.

REFERENCES

1. Dick RS, Steen EB, Detmer DE, editors. The computer-based patient record: an essential technology for health care, revised edition. Washington, DC: The National Academies Press; 1997.
2. Institute of Medicine (IOM). Crossing the quality chasm: a new health system for the 21st century. Washington, DC: The National Academies Press; 2001.
3. Mamykina L, Vawdrey DK, Stetson PD, et al. Clinical documentation: composition or synthesis? J Am Med Inform Assoc 2012;19(6):1025–31.
4. Institute of Medicine (IOM) Committee on Data Standards for Patient Safety. Key capabilities of an electronic health record system: letter report. Washington, DC: The National Academies Press; 2003.
5. Pantanowitz L, Tuthill JM, Balis UG. Pathology informatics: theory & practice. Chicago, IL: American Society of Clinical Pathologists Press; 2012.
6. Dolin RH, Alschuler L, Beebe C, et al. The HL7 clinical document architecture. J Am Med Inform Assoc 2001;8(6):552–69.
7. Bates DW, Leape LL, Cullen DJ, et al. Effect of computerized physician order entry and a team intervention on prevention of serious medication errors. JAMA 1998;280(15):1311–6.

8. Payne TH, Hoey PJ, Nichol P, et al. Preparation and use of preconstructed orders, order sets, and order menus in a computerized provider order entry system. J Am Med Inform Assoc 2003;10(4):322–9.

9. HealthIT.gov. Clinical Decision Support (CDS). Available at: http://www.healthit.gov/policy-researchers-implementers/clinical-decision-support-cds. Accessed July 8, 2014.

10. Tarczy-Hornoch P, Amendola L, Aronson SJ, et al. A survey of informatics approaches to whole-exome and whole-genome clinical reporting in the electronic health record. Genet Med 2013;15(10):824–32.

11. Yu P, Artz D, Warner J. Electronic health records (EHRs): supporting ASCO's vision of cancer care. Am Soc Clin Oncol Educ Book 2014;225–31.

12. HealthIT.gov. What is a patient portal? Available at: http://www.healthit.gov/providers-professionals/faqs/what-patient-portal. Accessed July 8, 2014.

13. HealthIT.gov. Health Information Exchange (HIE). Available at: http://www.healthit.gov/providers-professionals/health-information-exchange/what-hie. Accessed July 8, 2014.

Translational Bioinformatics and Clinical Research (Biomedical) Informatics

S. Joseph Sirintrapun, MD[a],*, Ahmet Zehir, PhD[b], Aijazuddin Syed, MS[b], JianJiong Gao, PhD[b], Nikolaus Schultz, PhD[b], Donavan T. Cheng, PhD[b]

KEYWORDS

- Translational informatics • Bioinformatics • Clinical research informatics
- Biomedical informatics • The Cancer Genome Atlas • TCGA • cBioPortal
- Cancer genomics

OVERVIEW OF TRANSLATIONAL BIOINFORMATICS AND CLINICAL RESEARCH (BIOMEDICAL) INFORMATICS

Translational bioinformatics and clinical research (biomedical) informatics are the primary domains related to informatics activities that support translational research. Although arguably distinct, clinical research (biomedical) informatics and translational bioinformatics are often used interchangeably. Translational bioinformatics focuses more specifically on the computational techniques in the areas of genetics, molecular biology, and systems biology.[1,2] By contrast, clinical research (biomedical) informatics involves the use of informatics in the discovery and management of new knowledge relating to health and disease.

Clinical research (biomedical) informatics uses computational techniques related to secondary research use of clinical information for understanding disease processes. These computational techniques span a wide set of interdisciplinary fields and encompass resources, devices, and methods that optimize the acquisition, storage, retrieval, transformation, and communication of clinical information.[1,2]

Driving both translational bioinformatics and clinical research (biomedical) informatics is the management and refinement of data: how data are captured, transmitted, processed, and conveyed into information in order to generate meaningful knowledge. How data are captured for translational bioinformatics begins after tissue acquisition and tissue processing, and uses advanced molecular techniques for data generation. How data are captured for clinical research (biomedical) informatics starts

This article originally appeared in Surgical Pathology Clinics, Volume 8, Issue 2, June 2015.
Disclosures: None.
[a] Department of Pathology, Memorial Sloan Kettering Cancer Center, 1275 York Avenue, New York, NY 10065, USA; [b] Memorial Sloan Kettering Cancer Center, 417 East 68th Street, New York, NY 10065, USA
* Corresponding author.
E-mail address: sirintrs@mskcc.org

Clin Lab Med 36 (2016) 153–181
http://dx.doi.org/10.1016/j.cll.2015.09.013
0272-2712/16/$ – see front matter © 2016 Elsevier Inc. All rights reserved.

with data compiled from health information systems (discussed in an article elsewhere in this issue).

One application of clinical research (biomedical) informatics is managing information related to clinical trials. Another application is linking large-scale DNA data banks with electronic medical record systems for discovery of genotype-phenotype associations.[3] Informatics of biospecimens and biorepositories also falls under the scope of clinical research (biomedical) informatics and is discussed briefly.

With biospecimens and biorepositories, there are immense infrastructural needs from information technology. Biospecimens and biorepositories must have associated quality clinical and pathology information with the specimens, which means efforts to determine which data elements to capture and easy mechanisms to associate and annotate samples. Optimal information systems can update whether studies have institutional review board approval using samples and associated clinical data elements. Moreover, there should be security maintenance and processes in place for de-identification of protected health information. Tools for de-identification could include an honest broker system, which maintains linkages between samples and clinical data elements through a third-party mediator.

Information systems for biospecimens and biorepositories should encompass operational logistics, such as inventory tracking, sample processing, storage, and distribution management. Sophisticated information systems have bar-coding systems to facilitate such operational logistics. Crucial are functionalities to document how specimens are acquired and collected. Other functionalities include refrigeration and location, specimen distribution, and usage and control user accessibility. Biospecimens and biorepositories are costly investments and there are pressures for such information systems to enable cost recovery measures.[4]

Creating an optimal information systems infrastructure for biospecimens and biorepositories has proved daunting. The cancer Biomedical Informatics Grid (caBIG) initiative began in 2004 to create an interoperable academic/commercial biomedical information system, built on community-driven, precompetitive open source standards for data exchange and interoperability in the cancer research enterprise. This initiative held hopes for widespread dissemination throughout the cancer community. The guiding principles of caBIG of open access, open development, and open source were appealing. The ideal vision for caBIG was to make large and diverse cancer research data sets sustainably available for analysis, integration, and mining. In doing so, caBIG would become the platform by which cancer researchers would access data and biospecimens across institutions to perform genomic analysis and to find and analyze clinical data. The caBIG initiative never achieved its ideal vision for multiple lengthy reasons which will not be discussed and, sadly, the caBIG initiative was retired.[5]

ILLUSTRATIVE EXAMPLES OF TRANSLATIONAL BIOINFORMATICS AND CLINICAL RESEARCH (BIOMEDICAL) INFORMATICS

This article details 3 projects that are hybrid applications of translational bioinformatics and clinical research (biomedical) informatics. The first is TCGA, the second is the cBioPortal for Cancer Genomics, the third is the MSKCC CVR system database; all were designed to facilitate insights into cancer biology and clinical/therapeutic correlations.

Part 1. The Cancer Genome Atlas

TCGA is a comprehensive and coordinated multi-institutional effort to create a detailed catalog, or atlas, of genetic mutations in cancer using advanced genome sequencing and translational bioinformatics associated with specific types of tumors to improve the prevention, diagnosis, and treatment of cancer. Its mission was to accelerate the understanding of the molecular basis of cancer through the application of genome analysis and characterization technologies.

TCGA began in 2006 as a pilot project funded by the National Cancer Institute (NCI) and National Human Genome Research Institute, both parts of the National Institutes of Health. Initially, TCGA focused on characterization of only 3 types of cancers but since has grown to at least 30 tumor types and many more subtypes.[6,7] The cancers were selected by TCGA because of their poor prognosis and overall public health impact. The power of the project is the quality of tissue acquisition. TCGA samples are consistent in their processing with extensive quality controls (QCs) in place. TCGA research network encompasses centers for genome characterization, protein characterization, and genomic data analysis centers, which enable the process for genomic discovery. TCGA network comprises scientists, bioinformaticians, bioethicists, doctors, nurses, and cancer advocates. The data generated includes gene expression, protein expression, DNA copy number alterations (CNAs), epigenomics (noninherited DNA modifications), and microRNAs (miRNAs), which are short RNAs that control gene expression. Genome sequencing centers perform exome (coding gene region) sequencing on all cases, with some cases selected for whole-genome (coding and noncoding gene region) sequencing. Genomic data analysis centers, through developed tools, analyze the vast amount of data generated in TCGA. This project has collected an unprecedented number of high-quality human cancer samples and matching normal controls to identify important genomic changes in the development of cancer.

The data are accessible for prepublication by (1) the Cancer Genomics Hub (https://cghub.ucsc.edu/), a database that houses lower-level sequence data and alignments, or (2) TCGA Data Portal (https://tcga-data.nci.nih.gov/tcga/tcgaHome2.jsp [**Fig. 1**]), where all other data, including some clinical information, are deposited. TCGA Data Portal hosts data sets that are queryable and include exome (variant analysis), single-nucleotide polymorphism (SNP), methylation, mRNA, miRNA, and de-identified patient clinical information from both tumor and matching normal samples (**Fig. 2**).[7] The data can also be accessed by several tools and portals developed by the genomic data analysis centers, including the Broad Firehose (http://gdac.broadinstitute.org/), Regulome Explorer (http://explorer.cancerregulome.org/), TumorPortal (http://cancergenome.broadinstitute.org/), University of California Santa Cruz Cancer Genomics Browser (https://genome-cancer.ucsc.edu/), Integrative Genomics Viewer (IGV) via the "Load from Server" option (http://www.broadinstitute.org/igv/), and cBioPortal for Cancer Genomics (http://cbioportal.org/) (discussed later).

Part 2. cBioPortal for Cancer Genomics

Large-scale cancer genomics projects, such as TCGA, generate overwhelming amounts of cancer genomics data from multiple different technical platforms, which increases the challenges of performing data integration, exploration, and analytics, especially for scientists without a computational background. There have been issues with making the large raw data sets more easily accessible and integrating the clinical information in a meaningful manner.[8–10]

The cBioPortal for Cancer Genomics (http://cbioportal.org [**Fig. 3**])[2] was specifically designed by MSKCC to lower the barriers of access to complex genomic data sets for cancer researchers who needed a rapid, intuitive, and high-quality interface to molecular profiles and clinical attributes from large-scale cancer genomics projects like TCGA. The simplifying concept of cBioPortal is to integrate multiple data types at

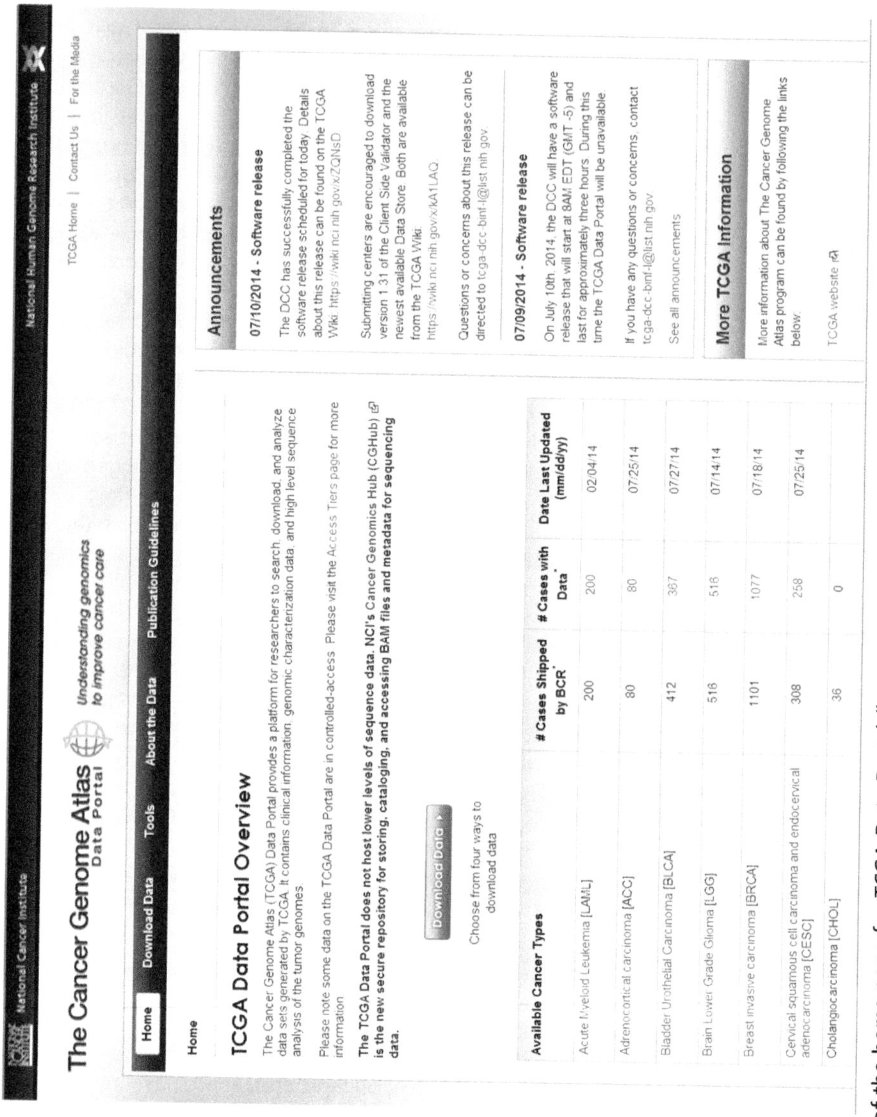

Fig. 1. Screenshot of the home page for TCGA Data Portal (https://tcga-data.nci.nih.gov/tcga/tcgaHome2.jsp).

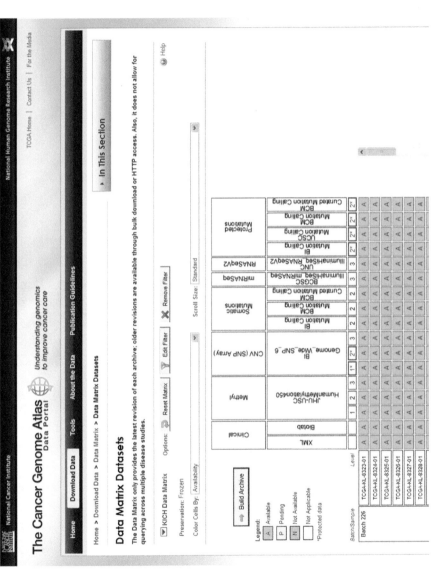

Fig. 2. Screenshot of a Web page in TCGA Data Portal for hosted data matrix/matrices of tumor samples. In addition to availability, data sets are queryable and include exome (variant analysis), SNP, methylation, mRNA, miRNA, and de-identified patient clinical information from both tumor and matching normal samples.

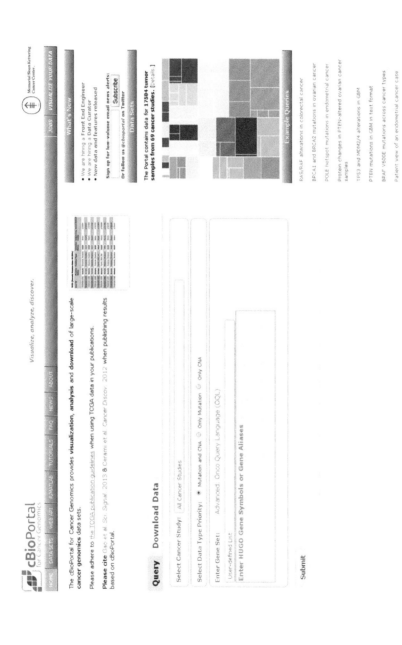

Fig. 3. Screenshot of the home page for the cBioPortal for Cancer Genomics (http://cbioportal.org).

the gene level and then query for the presence of specific biological events in each sample. Genomic data types integrated in cBioPortal include somatic mutations, DNA CNAs, mRNA and miRNA expression, DNA methylation, protein abundance, and phosphoprotein abundance, allowing users to query genetic alterations per gene and sample and test hypotheses regarding recurrence and genomic context of gene alteration events in specific cancers. This open platform bridges the translational bioinformatics of rich multidimensional cancer genomics data with the biomedical informatics of therapies and clinical trials to accelerate new biological insights and translation toward novel clinical applications.[8–10]

The data in cBioPortal come from more than 5000 tumor samples across 20 cancer studies. **Fig. 4** shows summarized results from a TCGA kidney renal clear cell carcinoma study in cBioPortal. Provisional data sets are continually updated as new TCGA cancer types are added. The cBioPortal facilitates the exploration of multidimensional cancer genomics data through better visualization and analysis across genes, samples, and data types. There are numerous tools in cBioPortal for evaluating biological processes and pathways in cancer. Gene alteration frequencies are comparable across multiple cancer studies. **Fig. 5** displays the gene alteration frequencies of the gene p53 in cBioPortal, where ovarian serous leads the list of cancer types with greater than 90% alteration frequency. **Fig. 6** shows the query from a provisional kidney renal papillary cell carcinoma study, which is selected for recurrently mutated genes. **Fig. 7** is from the same provisional kidney renal papillary cell carcinoma study, which displays selected genes from genomic regions with CNAs. Additional CNA details are viewable in cBioPortal through launching a Web start version of IGV. **Fig. 8** is the IGV showing the segmented copy number data of the provisional kidney renal clear cell carcinoma study with copy status of all queried genes.[8–10]

The OncoPrint of cBioPortal provides a concise and compact graphical summary of genomic alterations in genes involved in the selected cancer type. **Fig. 9** is the OncoPrint from the provisional kidney renal clear cell carcinoma study and shows that gene alterations in von Hippel-Lindau (VHL) comprise 54% of the cases but with the added insight that several of these cases show co-occurrence of alterations in genes PBRM1, SETD2, and BAP1. **Fig. 10** shows a mutation diagram for the PIK3CA gene from the same provisional kidney renal clear cell carcinoma study. Mutations and individual samples with PIK3CA mutations, as well as each mutation's number of occurrences in the Catalogue of Somatic Mutations in Cancer (COSMIC), are listed and annotated on PIK3CA protein domains.[8–10]

Information on co-occurrence (gene events occurring together) or mutual exclusivity (gene events not occurring together) is discoverable in cBioPortal. **Fig. 11** displays the statistics for co-occurrence and mutual exclusivity for genes from the provisional kidney renal clear cell carcinoma study. Through correlation plots, users have several different ways of visualizing discrete genetic events (CNAs or mutations) and continuous events, such as data regarding mRNA or protein abundance, or DNA methylation. **Fig. 12** shows the correlation plot between SETD2 mRNA expression and VHL mRNA expression, from the same provisional kidney renal clear cell carcinoma study. As shown in the OncoPrint in **Fig. 9**, a considerable number of cases show both mutations in SETD2 and VHL.[8–10]

The cBioPortal has the functionality for interactive analysis and visualization of altered networks. The networks consist of pathways and interactions from the Human Protein Reference Database,[11] Reactome,[12] NCI Pathway Interaction Database,[13] and the MSKCC Cancer Cell Map (http://cancer.cellmap.org), as derived from the open source Pathway Commons Project.[14] **Fig. 13** is the network view of altered

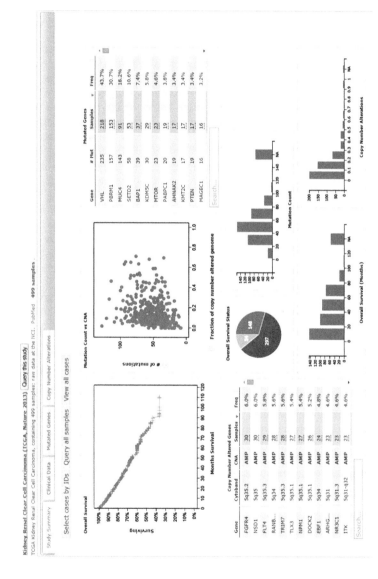

Fig. 4. Screenshot of a Web page in the cBioPortal, which illustrates how research studies are integrated and summarized visually. This Web page shows summarized results from a TCGA kidney renal clear cell carcinoma study correlating molecular information (ie, mutation count and CNAs) with clinical outcome data (ie, overall survival).

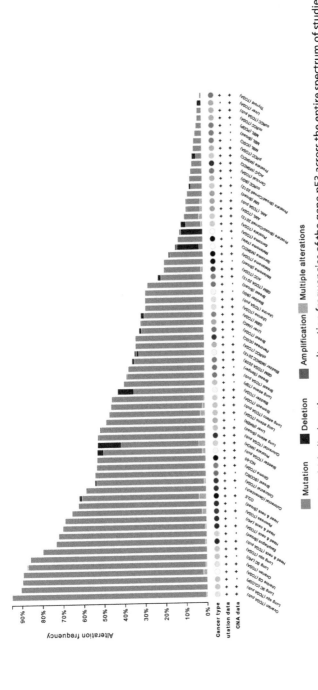

Fig. 5. Screenshot of a Web page in the cBioPortal, which displays the gene alteration frequencies of the gene p53 across the entire spectrum of studied tumor types. In this example, ovarian serous leads the list of cancer types with greater than 90% alteration frequency comprising almost entirely of mutations rather than deletions or amplifications.

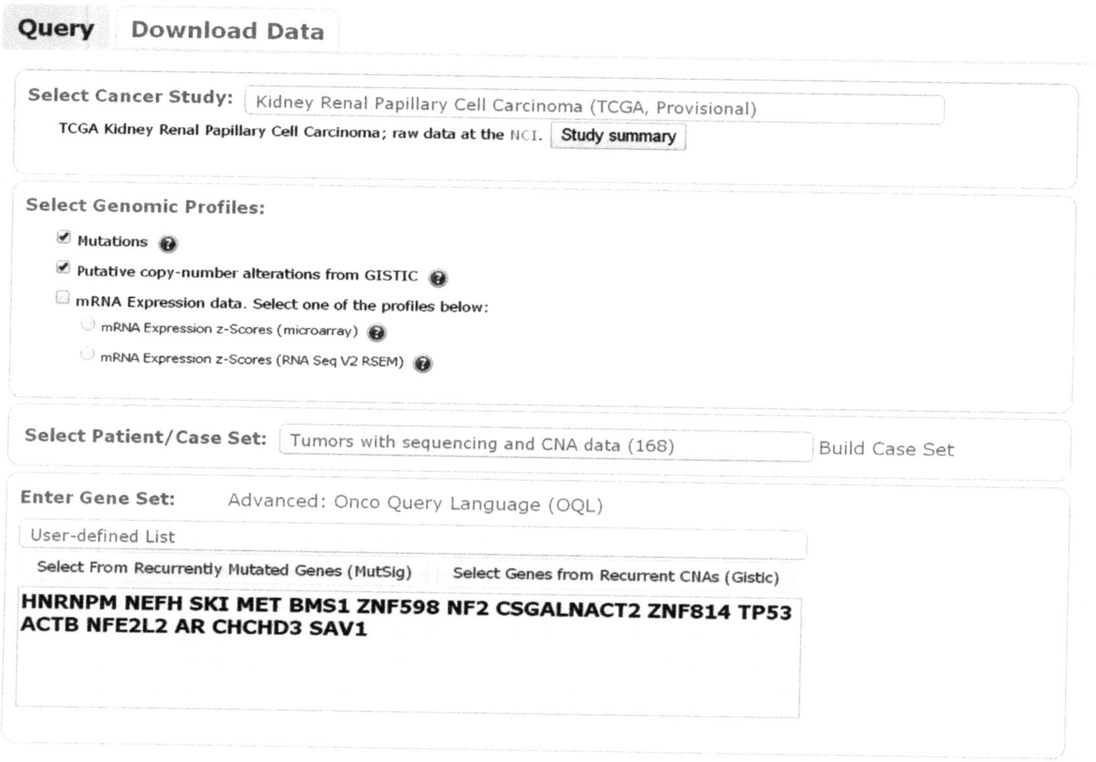

Fig. 6. Screenshot of a Web page in the cBioPortal illustrating the power of discovering recurrently mutated genes by tumor type. This example shows a query from a provisional kidney renal papillary cell carcinoma study, which is selected for recurrently mutated genes, such as MET.

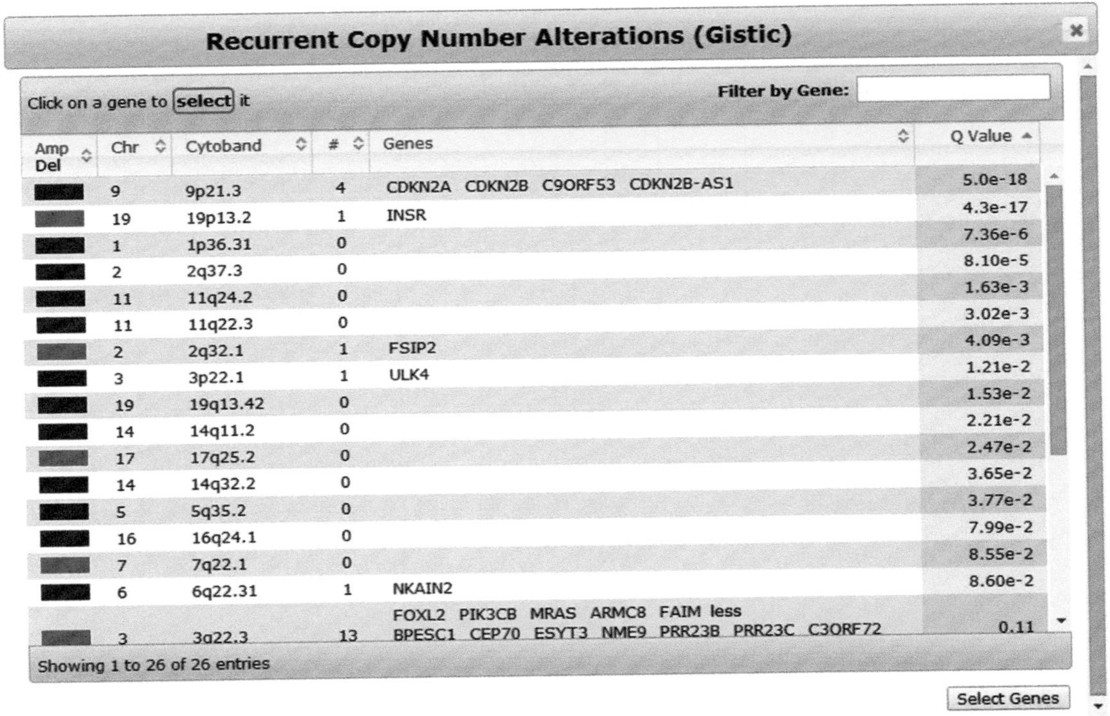

Recurrent Copy Number Alterations (Gistic)

Filter by Gene:

Click on a gene to [select] it

Amp Del	Chr	Cytoband	#	Genes	Q Value
	9	9p21.3	4	CDKN2A CDKN2B C9ORF53 CDKN2B-AS1	5.0e-18
	19	19p13.2	1	INSR	4.3e-17
	1	1p36.31	0		7.36e-6
	2	2q37.3	0		8.10e-5
	11	11q24.2	0		1.63e-3
	11	11q22.3	0		3.02e-3
	2	2q32.1	1	FSIP2	4.09e-3
	3	3p22.1	1	ULK4	1.21e-2
	19	19q13.42	0		1.53e-2
	14	14q11.2	0		2.21e-2
	17	17q25.2	0		2.47e-2
	14	14q32.2	0		3.65e-2
	5	5q35.2	0		3.77e-2
	16	16q24.1	0		7.99e-2
	7	7q22.1	0		8.55e-2
	6	6q22.31	1	NKAIN2	8.60e-2
	3	3q22.3	13	FOXL2 PIK3CB MRAS ARMC8 FAIM less BPESC1 CEP70 ESYT3 NME9 PRR23B PRR23C C3ORF72	0.11

Showing 1 to 26 of 26 entries

Select Genes

Fig. 7. Screenshot of a Web page in the cBioPortal illustrating the power of discovering selected genes from genomic regions with CNAs. This example is from the same provisional kidney renal papillary cell carcinoma study illustrated in **Fig. 6** and, for all described CNAs, the corresponding genes located in those regions are listed.

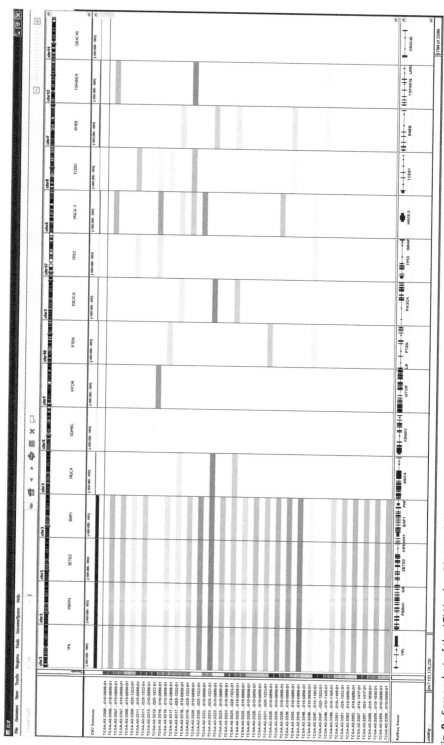

Fig. 8. Screenshot of the IGV in the cBioPortal showing the segmented copy number data of the provisional kidney renal clear cell carcinoma study with copy status of all queried genes.

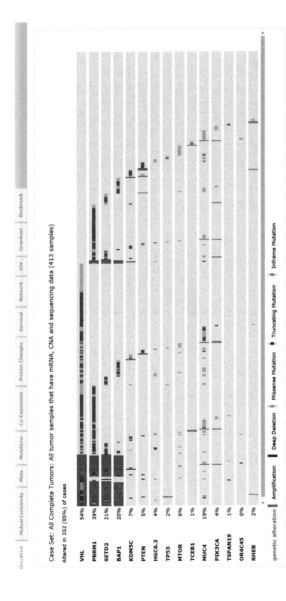

Fig. 9. Screenshot of an OncoPrint in the cBioPortal illustrating its power as a concise and compact graphical summary of genomic alterations in genes involved in the selected cancer type. This example is from the a provisional kidney renal clear cell carcinoma study and shows that gene alterations in VHL comprise 54% of the cases but with the added insight that several of these cases show co-occurrence of alterations in genes PBRM1, SETD2, and BAP1.

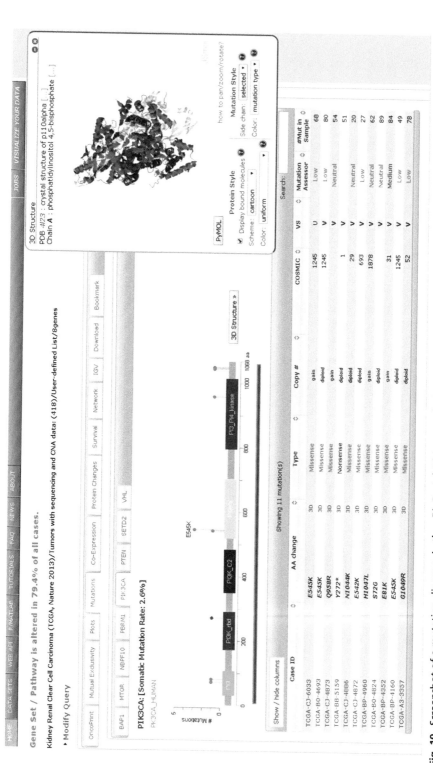

Fig. 10. Screenshot of a mutation diagram in the cBioPortal. This example illustrates the PIK3CA gene from the same provisional kidney renal clear cell carcinoma study illustrated in **Fig. 9**. Mutations and individual samples with PIK3CA mutations, as well as each mutation's number of occurrences in COSMIC, are listed and annotated on PIK3CA protein domains.

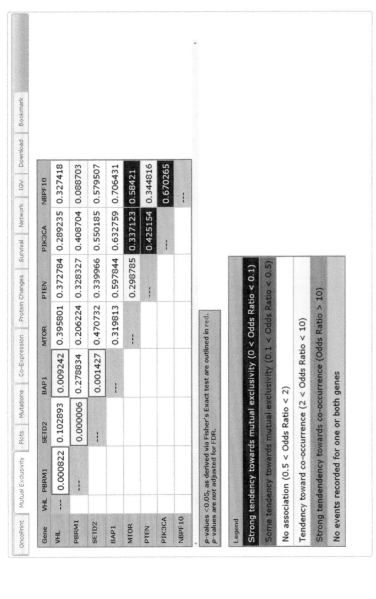

Fig. 11. Screenshot of a data matrix/matrices in the cBioPortal displaying the statistics for both co-occurrence and mutual exclusivity for genes. Through correlation plots, users have several different ways of visualizing discrete genetic events (CNAs or mutations) and continuous events, such as data regarding mRNA or protein abundance, or DNA methylation. This example is from the same provisional kidney renal clear cell carcinoma study illustrated in **Figs. 9** and **10**.

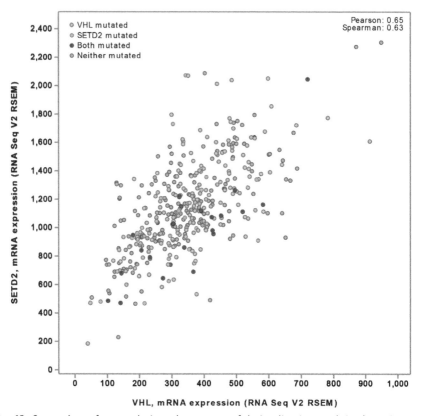

Fig. 12. Screenshot of a correlation plot, a powerful visualization tool, in the cBioPortal. This example is from the same provisional kidney renal clear cell carcinoma study illustrated in **Figs. 9–11**. The plot correlates SETD2 mRNA expression and VHL mRNA expression among samples. As shown in the OncoPrint in **Fig. 9**, a considerable number of cases show both mutations in SETD2 and VHL.

gene nodes, such as VHL derived from the provisional kidney renal clear cell carcinoma study.[8–10]

The biomedical informatics component of cBioPortal can display overall survival analysis and disease-free survival rates, if survival data are available. Overall survival and disease-free survival differences are computed between tumor samples that have at least one alteration in one of the query genes and tumor samples that do not. The results are displayed as Kaplan-Meier plots with P values from a log-rank test. **Fig. 14** shows the Kaplan-Meier plots focused on BAP1 from the provisional kidney renal clear cell carcinoma study and demonstrates a statistically significant difference in survival of cases with alterations of the BAP1 gene versus cases without alterations of the BAP1 gene.[8–10]

cBioPortal is currently being transitioned into a tool for the visualization genomic and clinical information of individual tumors (or even patients with multiple tumors), with the goal of its eventual use as a decision support system that can be used in patient treatment. Because tumor samples often have few driver mutations in a sea of background mutations, one key challenge is to identify the most likely driver events found in a tumor sample. cBioPortal does this by using prior information about genes

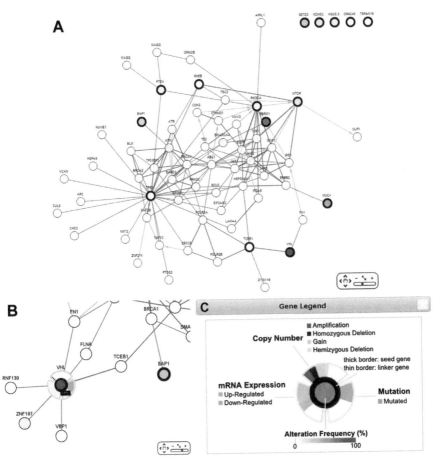

Fig. 13. Illustrates a network visualization tool of altered gene nodes in the cBioPortal. This example is from the same provisional kidney renal clear cell carcinoma study illustrated in **Figs. 9–12**. (*A*) The generalized network view of altered gene nodes. (*B*) Focuses on the VHL altered gene node and some interconnected gene nodes (ie, TCEB1). The BAP1 gene node is also within the proximity although not in direct connection with VHL. (*C*) Mouseover screenshot over the VHL altered gene node illustrating highly granular data, such as frequency of mutation, CNA, and mRNA expression.

and prior occurrence of specific mutations (eg, via the COSMIC database). cBioPortal also summarizes the key clinical annotation about a tumor sample, including basic demographic data of the patient, as well as stage and grade information about the tumor. For tumor samples from TCGA, links to the Cancer Digital Slide Archive are available, which allow fast and convenient viewing of histopathologic slides of all TCGA tumors. Furthermore, de-identified pathology reports can be viewed in PDF format for all TCGA samples. In the future, cBioPortal can be more tightly integrated with other clinical information systems in a hospital.

Part 3. Memorial Sloan Kettering Cancer Center—Clinical Variants and Results Database

The volume of genetic variants identified by clinical NGS assays poses a challenge in terms of variant visualization, classification, pathologist review, and sign-out.

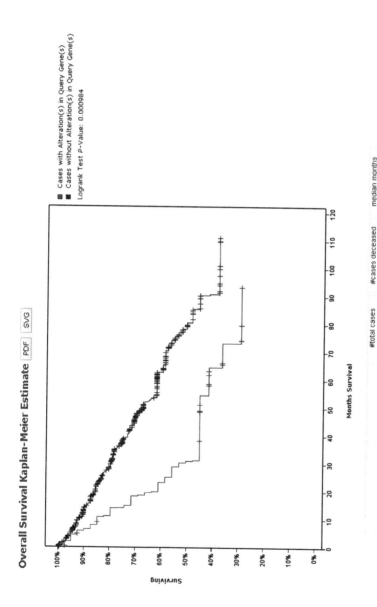

Fig. 14. Screenshot of a Kaplan-Meier visualization tool in the cBioPortal. This example focuses on BAP1 from the same provisional kidney renal clear cell carcinoma study illustrated in **Figs. 9–13** and demonstrates a statistically significant difference in survival of cases with alterations of the BAP1 gene versus cases without alterations of the BAP1 gene.

Guidelines from regulatory agencies, such as the College of American Pathologists or New York State Department of Health, impose additional requirements on tracking changes made during the sign-out process (passing or failing variant calls, editing of variant annotations, and so forth). From a longer-term perspective, a systematic organization of variant information and associated clinical and analysis metadata are essential to enable retrospective data mining and clinical phenotype correlative studies for biomarker discovery. To address these concerns the clinical bioinformatics group at MSKCC developed an in-house solution, called the CVR system, to organize and efficiently manage variants called by clinical NGS assays. The back-end CVR database is paired with an intuitive Web interface to streamline variant classification through manual review and sign-out.

The CVR system sits at the end of a clinical sequencing pipeline (shown in **Fig. 15**). The Clinical Laboratory Improvement Amendments–approved NGS tests at MSKCC are mainly targeted sequencing panels that vary in terms of assay technology (hybridization capture vs amplicon polymerase chain reaction), sequencing platform (Illumina vs Ion Torrent), scale (high throughput vs benchtop sequencer), and analysis pipeline. The CVR system is designed to be agnostic for the variables (listed previously) and accepts as its input a variant call format (VCF) or tab-delimited text file with a prespecified format. Metadata from a wet laboratory and analysis parts of the pipeline are managed by different laboratory information systems respectively: various procedures in the wet laboratory process are documented and tracked using an NGS-specialized laboratory information management system (LIMS), whereas metadata regarding sequencing QC and various analysis metrics are tracked using an in-house developed data management system (DMS). These metadata may be used to place variant calls into context during sign-out, and the CVR system uses API Web service calls to retrieve these metadata from the LIMS and DMS, for presentation in the sign-out Web interface.

Use cases for the clinical variants and results system

The development of the CVR system was motivated by the following use cases.

Development of a data warehousing solution As NGS testing scales up in a clinical laboratory, the results of different runs of various tests may be stored in an ad hoc manner in scattered locations, complicating data backup and subsequent information retrieval. The authors desire a central storage system where all molecular pathology diagnostic test results can be systematically housed and looked up in subsequent queries.

Improving how change history is tracked Pathologists may reject variant calls based on experience and prior knowledge or even edit the cDNA and amino acid annotations for a given mutation to be compliant with Human Genome Variation Society (HGVS) standards. These changes should be memorialized in a database, so there is accountability for differences between variants called by the pipeline and variants that are entered into a patient's pathology report.

Facilitating the sign-out process Depending on the size of the targeted sequencing panel, whether a patient matched normal is used, or filters set in the data analysis pipeline, NGS tests may return on the order of tens to thousands of variants. Reviewing each variant during sign-out by browsing for the appropriate alignment file and manually entering variant coordinates is a time-consuming process that cannot be scaled to large volumes. An automated solution for quick visualization of genomic data and variant calls is needed for facilitating sign-out of NGS test results.

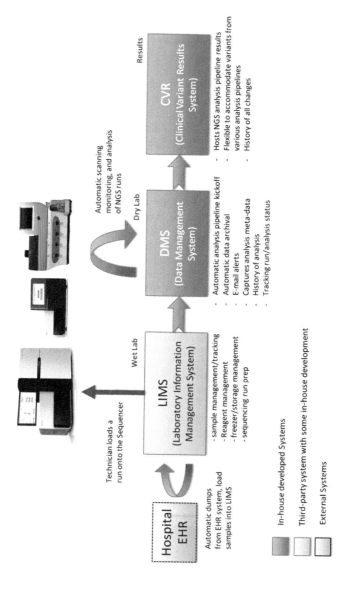

Fig. 15. Schematic of the clinical sequencing pipeline at MSKCC. The CVR system sits at the end of a clinical sequencing pipeline.

Providing a start-to-finish dashboard view of laboratory operations Many steps in the NGS pipeline (sample QC, wet laboratory workflow, and analysis steps) can affect the quality of the final variant calling output. To streamline and optimize processes and turnaround time, laboratory directors should have access to a laboratory operations dashboard, which integrates collected metadata from various parts of the pipeline (LIMS and DMS) and is capable of correlating various metrics against pipeline output (CVR).

Implementation
Database schema The underlying schema of the MSKCC CVR database is based on the central idea that a set of variant calls is the product of an analysis pipeline configuration applied to the sequencing output for a given sample. Changes to either the pipeline configuration or sequencing result for a sample can alter the variant calling output, and it is essential to capture metadata on the pipeline, sample, and variant result levels to ensure provenance (**Fig. 16**). Examples of analysis pipeline metadata include time and date information, file system locations, pipeline versions, pipeline configurations, identifiers for bioinformatics analysts kicking off the pipeline, and so forth. Most of these metadata are already tracked by the DMS system, so the CVR system merely stores a DMS entity identification (ID), which it can use to retrieve the full set of metadata associated with the pipeline run from the DMS, using a Web service call if necessary. The CVR recognizes that a single patient may have multiple samples sequenced in various batches, which may differ in terms of sample type (ie, primary vs metastasis vs normal vs liquid biopsy), processing method (ie, formalin-fixed paraffin-embedded vs fresh vs frozen), or even purpose of inclusion within the sequenced batch (ie, clinical sequencing vs clinical validation vs translational research). Similar to the analysis pipeline metadata, most of the sample and patient information can be retrieved from the wet laboratory LIMS via a Web service call, so the CVR stores an LIMS entity ID instead of replicating most of this information. The atomic data unit within the CVR can thus be thought of as a DMS entity–LIMS entity data unit pair, which allows flexibility for situations where the same sample is put through various iterations of analysis or if the same analysis pipeline is repeatedly applied to multiple samples.

The CVR entity data unit (analysis pipeline sample pair) is linked to data tables describing various classes of mutation events (eg, point mutations [single nucleotide variations], indels, CNAs [whole-gene and partial/intragenic events], and structural rearrangements [translocations, tandem duplications, and inversions]). Similar to a reference SNP identifier (rsID) in the Single Nucleotide Polymorphism Database (dbSNP), or a COSMIC ID, each mutation observed is given a distinct CVR variant ID to facilitate queries of mutation prevalence (ie, the most commonly observed mutation in a given tumor type). The schema is flexible to accommodate both somatic and germline variants, but germline mutations are deliberately stored in a separate set of data tables, which can be access regulated depending on the level of patient consent.

Each set of data tables is provisioned by corresponding history tables, which maintain a detailed history of changes to table content, along with the ID of the user responsible for the changes. Data tables may be reverted to a previous version to undo changes, if necessary. In particular, individual variants may be deemed low-confidence or false-positive results (artifacts) over the course of manual review and sign-out. These variants are not deleted from the data tables but rather annotated with different flags under variant status: pending, rejected, and signed out. User IDs responsible for changes are not only tracked for accounting purposes but also

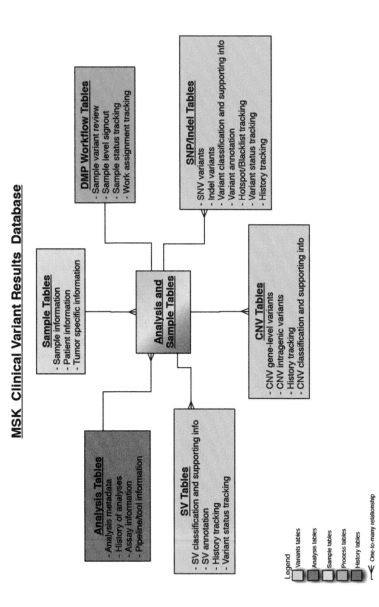

Fig. 16. Relational schematic underlying the MSKCC CVR database.

managed, so that only certain users within specified user groups have modification privileges. The codebase for various modules regulating the CVR system is complex—the back-end for the database interactions is written in Python, and SQLAlchemy is used to abstract the underlying server technology.

Web portal The Python Web development framework, Flask, is used for Web application development. The interface is supplemented with several JavaScript libraries to facilitate better usability and is hosted through an Apache server. A Web interface allows users to view variants using the IGV directly through hyperlinks, update clinical and diagnostic information, and automatically generate clinical reports reflecting assessments made during sign-out.

Fig. 17 shows the index page of the CVR Web portal that a pathologist sees when logging on and selecting a diagnostic test to sign out. In this example, Memorial Sloan Kettering–Integrated Mutation Profiling of Actionable Cancer Targets (MSK-IMPACT) is chosen, a hybridization capture-based targeted sequencing panel for 341 cancer-related genes. Different batches, or clinical runs, are listed as rows and can be expanded to display all sequenced samples within a given batch. Samples are colored based on their status: blue for pending (awaiting sign-out), yellow for sign-out complete but clinical report not generated, and green for sign-out complete and clinical report submitted to the pathology electronic health records database (ie, Cerner CoPath).

On selecting a particular sample, a pathologist is brought to a new tab in the Web portal, where salient patient and sample information is displayed up front (**Fig. 18**), including patient first and last names, whether a matched normal was used for somatic mutation calling, medical record number, sample accession number, and gender and depth of sequencing coverage for the sample (usually >500× for MSK-IMPACT). Fields, such as tumor type, sample type (primary vs metastasis), and tumor purity (ie, usually 20% or higher—a QC requirement for testing), are editable at the point of sign-out; they are populated with suggested content based on information imported from other databases, but pathologists are required to check, confirm, and/or edit these fields at sign-out.

The mutations detected are listed below the patient and sample information (**Fig. 19**). Pathologists are able to filter and search for mutations in a given gene of interest by typing into a Google-style search field. The listed mutation locations are a set of hyperlinks to IGV session XML files, which, on clicking, direct the user to the specific mutated locus in the sample alignment file (BAM file) using IGV. Mouseovers of the Human Genome Organisation (HUGO) gene symbols listed in the table bring up additional information from other cancer genome annotation resources, such as My Cancer Genome. The table also contains coverage and sequencing statistics for each variant call, including sequencing depth at the location of the variant, number of mutant reads, and mutant allele frequency in both the tumor and comparator normal. Pathologists are able to edit cDNA and amino acid annotations to ensure compliance with HGVS standards by clicking on an "edit" button and "drop" variants that they consider low confidence or artifacts (**Fig. 20**). In addition, pathologists can memorialize their rationale for editing or dropping variants as free text comments using the portal interface, by typing into the "comments" field and clicking "save."

Analytics
Applications pulling data from the LIMS, DMS, and CVR databases allow laboratory directors to monitor various aspects of laboratory operations. For instance, because the sample, analysis pipeline, and mutation results are consolidated in their respective

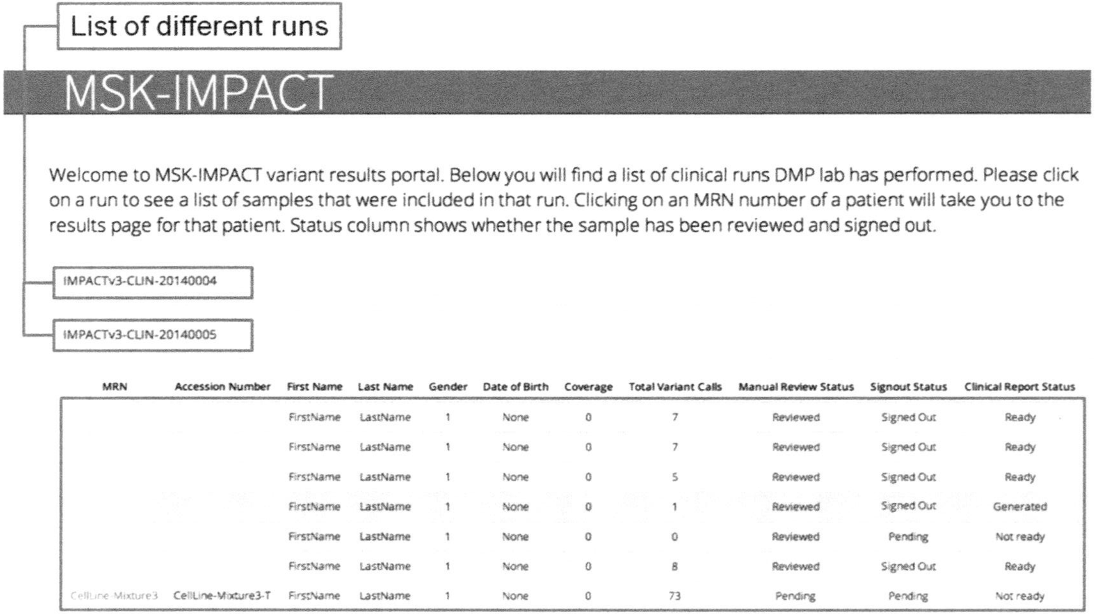

List of different runs

MSK-IMPACT

Welcome to MSK-IMPACT variant results portal. Below you will find a list of clinical runs DMP lab has performed. Please click on a run to see a list of samples that were included in that run. Clicking on an MRN number of a patient will take you to the results page for that patient. Status column shows whether the sample has been reviewed and signed out.

IMPACTv3-CLIN-20140004

IMPACTv3-CLIN-20140005

MRN	Accession Number	First Name	Last Name	Gender	Date of Birth	Coverage	Total Variant Calls	Manual Review Status	Signout Status	Clinical Report Status
		FirstName	LastName	1	None	0	7	Reviewed	Signed Out	Ready
		FirstName	LastName	1	None	0	7	Reviewed	Signed Out	Ready
		FirstName	LastName	1	None	0	5	Reviewed	Signed Out	Ready
		FirstName	LastName	1	None	0	1	Reviewed	Signed Out	Generated
		FirstName	LastName	1	None	0	0	Reviewed	Pending	Not ready
		FirstName	LastName	1	None	0	8	Reviewed	Signed Out	Ready
CellLine-Mixture1	CellLine-Mixture3-T	FirstName	LastName	1	None	0	73	Pending	Pending	Not ready

Fig. 17. Screenshot of the index page of the CVR Web portal, which represents the pathologist workspace environment for interpretation of the clinical sequencing pipeline at MSKCC that a pathologist sees when logging on and selecting a diagnostic test to sign out. This example shows the MSK-IMPACT test, a hybridization capture-based targeted sequencing panel for 341 cancer-related genes.

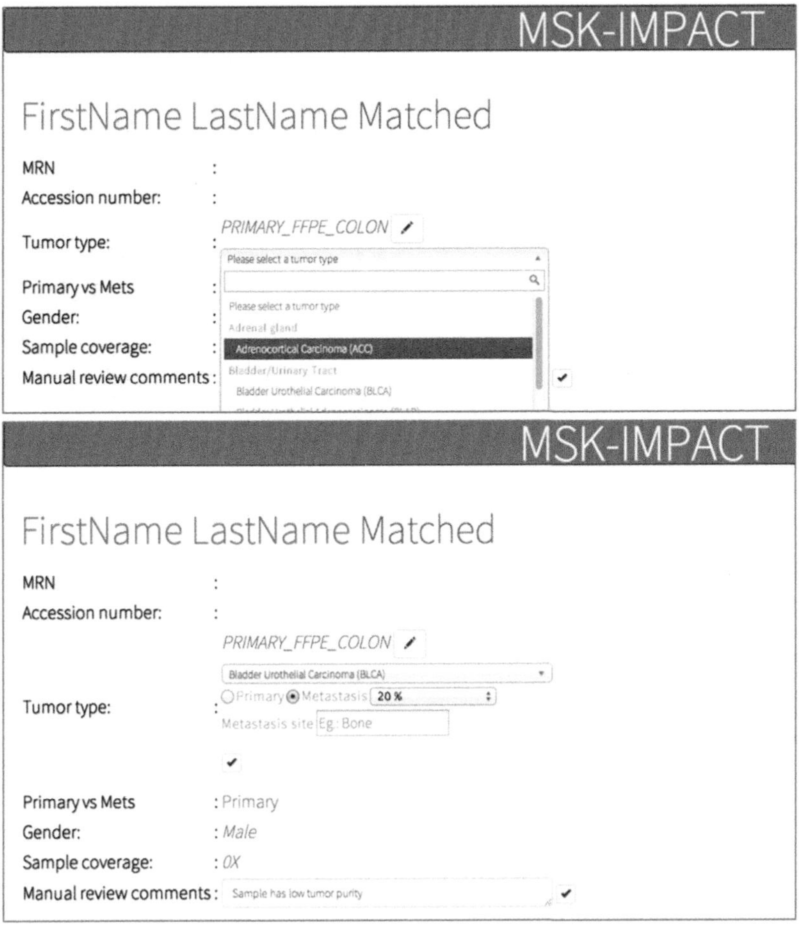

Fig. 18. Screenshot of subsequent tab from the index page in the CVR Web portal, on selecting a particular sample. The salient patient and sample information is displayed up front.

databases, directors can ask which solid tumor service or disease management team has been ordering the most number of diagnostic tests on a month-to-month basis (**Fig. 21**). Users can also perform high-level analytics to identify correlations between wet laboratory QC metrics (input DNA yield, tumor purity, library concentration, and so forth) and variant calling output, which may help identify thresholds or criteria on these metrics, below which a sample is sent to alternative means of diagnostic testing.

Extension to molecular diagnostic assays in general
The CVR database was initially designed as a warehouse for results of clinical NGS assays, but its underlying database schema is flexible enough to be extended to storing the results of non-NGS–based molecular diagnostic tests (eg, Sanger sequencing, fluorescence in situ hybridization, and short or tandem repeat assays). Depending on the assay output, additional variant tables may need to be created to handle the different classes of mutations called. Finally, to include non-NGS diagnostic assays under the same umbrella of DMSs developed for NGS tests, it is likely that the LIMS and DMS systems would also need to be extended to manage non-NGS tests. This

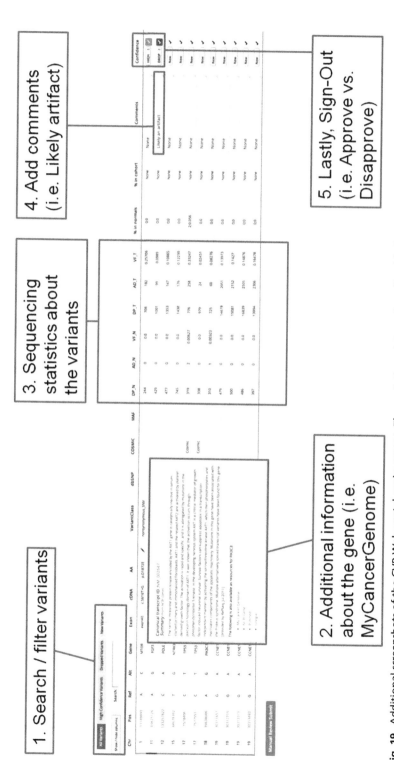

Fig. 19. Additional screenshots of the CVR Web portal environment. The mutations detected are listed below the patient and sample information and the pathologist is able to filter and search for mutations in a given gene of interest by typing into a Google-style search field. The listed mutation locations are a set of hyperlinks to IGV session XML files, which, on clicking, direct the user to the specific mutated locus in the sample alignment file (BAM file) using IGV.

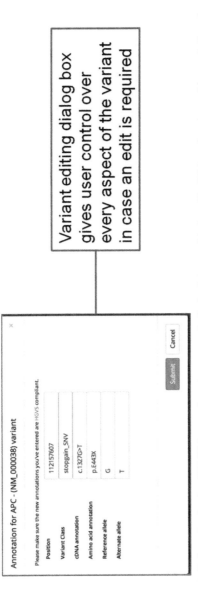

Fig. 20. Annotate/edit function in the CVR Web portal environment. Pathologists are able to edit cDNA and amino acid annotations to ensure compliance with HGVS standards by clicking on an "edit" button and "drop" variants that they consider "low confidence" or artifacts.

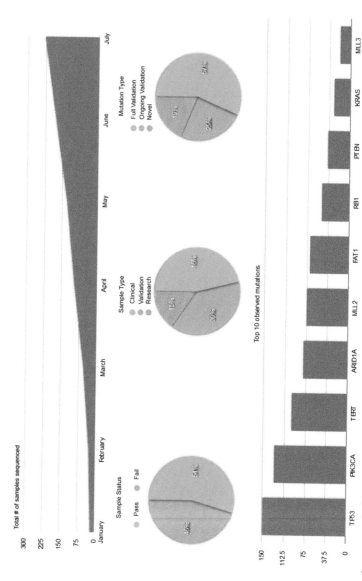

Fig. 21. Integrated summary dashboard in the CVR Web portal environment. Leverages the power of applications pulling data from the LIMS, DMS, and CVR databases to allow laboratory directors to monitor various aspects of laboratory operations and query for answers to administrative/operational questions, such as which solid tumor service or disease management team has been ordering the most number of diagnostic tests, on a month-to-month basis.

may be more challenging for the DMS system than for the LIMS, because the LIMS is assay agnostic and certain assays may be run with vendor-proprietary software that is not amenable to integration with an in-house developed analysis pipeline management system. In such cases, workarounds (ie, considering vendor software systems as a black box) may be necessary.

REFERENCES

1. Clinical research informatics. Available at: http://www.amia.org/applications-informatics/clinical-research-informatics. Accessed July 9, 2014.
2. Pantanowitz L, Tuthill JM, Balis UG. Pathology informatics: theory & practice. Chicago, IL: American Society of Clinical Pathologists Press; 2012.
3. Ritchie MD, Denny JC, Crawford DC, et al. Robust replication of genotype-phenotype associations across multiple diseases in an electronic medical record. Am J Hum Genet 2010;86(4):560–72.
4. Dash RC, Robb JA, Booker DL, et al. Biospecimens and biorepositories for the community pathologist. Arch Pathol Lab Med 2012;136(6):668–78.
5. Digital capabilities to accelerate research. Available at: https://cabig.nci.nih.gov/. Accessed August 1, 2014.
6. Wikipedia. The Cancer genome atlas. Available at: http://en.wikipedia.org/wiki/The_Cancer_Genome_Atlas#cite_note-2. Accessed July 9, 2014.
7. Atlas, T.C.G. Program overview. Available at: http://cancergenome.nih.gov/abouttcga/overview. Accessed July 9, 2014.
8. cBioPortal. Available at: http://www.cbioportal.org/public-portal/. Accessed August 1, 2014.
9. Cerami E, Gao J, Dogrusoz U, et al. The cBio cancer genomics portal: an open platform for exploring multidimensional cancer genomics data. Cancer Discov 2012;2(5):401–4.
10. Gao J, Aksoy BA, Dogrusoz U, et al. Integrative analysis of complex cancer genomics and clinical profiles using the cBioPortal. Sci Signal 2013;6(269):pl1.
11. Keshava Prasad TS, Goel R, Kandasamy K, et al. Human Protein Reference Database–2009 update. Nucleic Acids Res 2009;37(Database issue):D767–72.
12. Matthews L, Gopinath G, Gillespie M, et al. Reactome knowledgebase of human biological pathways and processes. Nucleic Acids Res 2009;37(Database issue):D619–22.
13. Schaefer CF, Anthony K, Krupa S, et al. PID: the Pathway Interaction Database. Nucleic Acids Res 2009;37(Database issue):D674–9.
14. Cerami EG, Gross BE, Demir E, et al. Pathway Commons, a web resource for biological pathway data. Nucleic Acids Res 2011;39(Database issue):D685–90.

Training in Informatics
Teaching Informatics in Surgical Pathology

Lewis Allen Hassell, MD*, Kenneth E. Blick, PhD

KEYWORDS

- Informatics • Surgical pathology • Milestones • Problem-based learning
- Competency

OVERVIEW

What, me worry?
—Alfred E. Neuman

The ability to stand calm and "keep your head when all about you are losing theirs" ("If," Rudyard Kipling) can come from 1 of 2 sources: (1) the confidence born of solid preparation, study, drill, and experience under stress or (2) the nonchalance derived from some combination of ignorance and apathy, oft epitomized by the hero of *Mad* magazine (quoted previously). For practicing pathologists today, and for the soon-to-be practitioners of that art and craft, the latter approach to the issues surrounding the informatics field is a recipe for more than comic-book disaster. But the challenge has been centered on how to form the foundation of knowledge and integrate the kind of drill and experience within the protected environs of a training program that can formulate the former kind of calm. The prior articles in this volume and an extensive literature on this topic have made the case for the essential skills of pathology informatics (PI), and most practices currently have at least one and often many staff members using these to some degree or another. This article aims to describe a less-than-haphazard or nonchalant approach to acquiring and instilling those essential information technology (IT) skills and knowledge within the context of existing learning models and training programs. This approach entails a review of learning and teaching approaches in the existing graduate medical education setting (residencies and to a lesser degree fellowships) and the postgraduate environment.

This article originally appeared in Surgical Pathology Clinics, Volume 8, Issue 2, June 2015.
Department of Pathology, University of Oklahoma Health Sciences Center, BMSB 451, 940 Stanton L Young Boulevard, Oklahoma City, OK 73104, USA
* Corresponding author.
E-mail address: Lewis-hassell@ouhsc.edu

Clin Lab Med 36 (2016) 183–197
http://dx.doi.org/10.1016/j.cll.2015.09.014
0272-2712/16/$ – see front matter © 2016 Elsevier Inc. All rights reserved.

THE WHAT—CURRICULUM CONTENT

Residency education generally, and pathology specifically, has migrated from a time-based apprenticeship model validated by a highly knowledge-based examination to an approach strongly emphasizing specific demonstrated competencies.[1] This follows a trend toward competency emphasis across medical education generally but most strongly manifests in graduate medical training.[2,3] Pathology has not been a laggard in this move and, accordingly, used the opportunity to flesh out learning and skill needs in an array of areas beyond conventional medical knowledge of diseases and morphologies to include the growing areas of molecular diagnostics, genomics, laboratory management, and informatics. The detailed and comprehensive exposition of the learning objectives and skill areas in informatics was developed soon after the Accreditation Council for Graduate Medical Education (ACGME) introduced its 6 competency areas by Henricks and colleagues[4] working in collaboration with the Association for Pathology Informatics (API). Significantly, their approach carefully divided the knowledge areas essential to pathologists along with the applications of that understanding in common use from the informatics proficiencies or skill sets to be sought or demonstrated by the learners.

The Pathology Milestones Project codified this effort on a broad scale into an array of competency statements and descriptors that capture different levels of competency within each area. Looking at the Milestones superficially, it might be concluded that only 1 category (Systems-Based Practice [SBP] competency 7—Informatics: Explains, Discusses, Classifies, and Applies Clinical Informatics) is pertinent to the topic of this article.[5] But in reality, a more comprehensive and inclusive definition, such as might be drawn from a review of model curricula of informatics, reveals that a host of other competency statements within the Milestones document also has direct bearing on informatics knowledge and skills (**Table 1**).

This question of what PI is and, therefore, what may need to be taught to enable practitioners to be proficient in it's essential uses is a nontrivial one—although neither is it a particularly foreign debate. Pathology has always fostered camps of *lumpers* and *splitters*, who look at their fields of investigation differently, broadly and narrowly, respectively (see, for example, Tischler[6]) Seen broadly, PI encompasses an extensive knowledge and skill base that enables effectively collecting, storing, managing, maintaining, retrieving, analyzing, interpreting, and creating data pertinent to the care of patients who come under the care of a laboratory or a caregiver using a laboratory. The required skill set may include the management of the metadata of the laboratory itself, the medical literature, or other data sets pertinent to 1 or more of the these activities. A more narrow definition is that proposed by Gabril and Yousef[7] of "using highly advanced technologies to improve patient diagnosis or management," which they largely distilled down to the use of current advanced tools in imaging and image transmission along with data mining. Although the authors acknowledge that a majority of "advanced practitioners" of PI will be using and managing those tools, the reality is that the broad definition means that every pathologist must have certain PI skills and knowledge to be effective. It is also the more broad definition that has formed the foundation of several recent solid textbooks in PI. **Table 2** summarizes the core curriculum content for residency-level training.

This curriculum content has recently been integrated into a tool for use by training programs, the result of joint work of the Association of Pathology Chairs (APC), College of American Pathologists (CAP), and API. This project and tool, Pathology Informatics Essentials for Residents (PIER), meshes well with the Milestone SBP7 and provides a graduated progression corresponding to the competency levels desired from residents during each year of training (**Fig. 1**). This program does not, however, attempt to address the broad needs (captured in **Table 1**) in the many other Milestones with PI components, perhaps with the recognition that a core understanding has many spin-off effects applied to other areas of training.

Looking further at postresidency-level training, either in a formal fellowship or a continuing medical education context, **Table 3** outlines recommended added content.[8] Training experience at this level, however, becomes more project driven and experiential, leading to a portfolio of competencies based on successful performance and endeavor in solving informatics-based problems.

THE HOW—METHOD(S) OF TEACHING/LEARNING PATHOLOGY INFORMATICS

Unlike much of the training in anatomic pathology, which is individual patient case based and more easily organized around ongoing clinical materials, acquiring skills in PI cannot be readily compartmentalized into a single rotation of a few weeks (**Box 1**). Although the content and knowledge have been organized for transmission via texts[9,10] or lectures on an intermittent or even condensed basis and presented in a case-study format using more or less real situations, these approaches often fall short of producing the level of competency required in the SBP7 and other competencies listed in **Table 1**. Nevertheless, such efforts help build IT vocabulary and create the foundation from which more applied skills can be developed. The PIER approach also recognizes that although some content can be encapsulated into time blocks, the higher-level applications can best be acquired using a variety of approaches, including journals, texts, mentors, and project-based experiences.

Several model programs have published their approach to laying this foundation. For example, Dr Pantanowitz's group has applied the crowd-sourcing power of a wiki to maintain the core content in their informatics block.[11] This approach builds on their prior efforts via a "virtual rotation"[12] and on efforts in other aspects of medical training where expertise may be otherwise difficult to access. Students can also benefit from these shared responsibilities.[13] This method of teaching/learning seems highly effective as witnessed by outcomes showing significantly higher levels of student IT performance based on assessments after implementation. This success is due in large part to the greater level of student engagement in the learning process. The old adage, "see, do, teach," is followed to a much greater degree as the students interact with the existing material and critique and refine it to make the content more meaningful on a personal basis.

PI is also a core competency area in the Laboratory Management University offering created by the American Pathology Foundation and the American Society for Clinical Pathology, launched in 2013.[14] This curriculum uses a blended learning model of online and live sessions coupled with a virtual community and offers numerous courses in each of the core management competency areas, including IT. The offerings are taught and developed by leaders in the field and geared to both the resident-level and also a new-in-practice leadership audience. This curriculum content is also being mapped to the Milestones (R. Weiss, personal communication, 2014) for use in developing other tools to assist program directors. The authors' experience in using these tools in resident education has been that the courses provide a solid foundation for discussion of a variety of topics, including PI; these discussions prompt potential topics for further competency development through chartered projects or other associated learning activities. Also, the authors have often coupled the discussions with evaluation of real and simulated case studies and have observed that trainees learn

Table 1
Pathology Milestones with significant informatics components

Milestone	Guiding Competency	Specific Statement	Pathology Informatics Curriculum Area
PC1	Analyzes, appraises, formulates, generates, and effectively reports consultations	Understands and applies EMR to obtain added clinical information (L1)	LIS; clinical information systems
PC2	Interpretation and reporting: analyzes data, appraises, formulates, and generates effective and timely reports	Proficient in using health care records and clinical information to develop a limited and focused differential diagnosis (L5)	Clinical information systems; data analysis; search engines
PC3	Interpretation and diagnosis: demonstrates knowledge and practices interpretation and analysis to formulate diagnoses	Analyzes complex cases, integrates literature, and prepares a full consultative written report with comprehensive review of medical records (L4)	Databases; search engines; data analysis
PC4	Reporting: analyzes data, appraises, formulates, and generates effective and timely reports	Able to complete synoptic report accurately (L4) Keeps current with evolving standards of synoptic reporting (L5)	Databases; data analysis
PC5	Procedure: surgical pathology grossing—demonstrates attitudes, knowledge, and practices that enable proficient performance of gross examination (analysis and appraisal of findings, synthesis and assembly, and reporting)	Produces reports that contain all the necessary information for patient management; edits transcribed reports effectively (L3)	Fundamentals of computing; word processing, databases
MK1	Diagnostic knowledge: demonstrates attitudes, knowledge, and practices that incorporate evidence-based medicine and promote lifelong learning	Performs scientific literature review and investigation of clinical cases to inform patient care (evidence-based medicine) and improve diagnostic knowledge of pathology (L3)	Databases, search engines, data analysis
SBP1	Patient safety: demonstrates attitudes, knowledge, and practices that contribute to patient safety	Explores other resources, such as EMR and radiology (L2) Trouble-shoots patient safety issues (including preanalytical, analytical, and postanalytical), as needed, without supervision (L4)	Laboratory and clinical information systems; connectivity; interfaces and networks Data analysis, graphic tools; data protection and backup

SPB2	Laboratory management: regulatory and compliance	Understands coding and the need to document appropriately in reports (L3) Uses best practices for billing compliance (L5) Understand and apply/teaches others policies and procedures in PHI as defined by HIPAA (L2/L3/L4)	Security, privacy, and confidentiality of laboratory data
SBP3	Laboratory management: resource utilization	Recognizes different budget types (L2) Develops and manages a laboratory budget (L5)	Fundamentals of computing; spreadsheets
SBP4	Laboratory management: quality, risk management, and laboratory safety	Interprets quality data and charts and trends (L3) Has completed a quality improvement project (L4) Utilizes continuous improvement tools, such as lean and Six Sigma (L5)	Databases, user interface; spreadsheets
SBP5	Laboratory management: test utilization	Organizes basic data for utilization review (L2) Able to create charts and graphs that demonstrate utilization patterns (L4) Demonstrates a broad portfolio of analyses for UR in complex scenarios and team management to drive change in areas both within and outside of the department (L5)	Presentation graphics; spreadsheets
SBP6	Laboratory management: technology assessment	Able to perform a cost-benefit analysis (L3) Participates in new instrument and test selection, verification, implementation and validation (including reference range analysis) (L4)	Data analysis; spreadsheets
SBP7	Informatics		See text and **Fig. 1**
PBLI1	Recognition of errors and discrepancies	Participates in RCA (L3)	Various
PROF1	Licensing, certification, examinations, credentialing	Begins assembling portfolio of experiences, including case log and participation in administrative tasks (L2)	Fundamentals of computing; database
ICS2	Interdepartmental and health care clinical team interactions	Prepares and presents cases at multidisciplinary conferences (L3)	Image management; presentation graphics

Abbreviations: EMR, electronic medical record; HIPAA, Health Insurance Portability and Accountability Act; ICS, interpersonal communication skills; L, level; MK, medical knowledge; PBL, practice-based learning; PC, patient care; PHI, personal health information; PROF, professionalism; RCA, root cause analysis; SBP, systems based practice; UR, utilization of resources.

Table 2
Residency-level curriculum for pathology informatics

Core Area	Terms and Concepts	Applications
Computing fundamentals	Hardware Software Networks Internet related	Storage selection System performance Interfaces Languages Architecture
LIS	LIS components Data standards System management Software customization	Critical feature selection Implementation process RFP process Integration Service model selection Trade-offs between types
Data analysis	Databases Transactions Analytics	Expert systems Architecture and type Data mining
Security, privacy, and confidentiality	HIPAA Audits Firewalls Encryption	Selection of security methods Data backup options Compliance planning
Regulatory issues	Audits and standards Compliance planning Accreditation bodies	Inspection planning Documentation Risk avoidance
Digital imaging and telepathology	Pixel, resolution, bits Compression Image analysis Storage Streaming	Scanning options Storage planning Clinical solutions Integration
Additional technologies	Voice recognition Artificial intelligence -Omics Multiplex data streams	

Abbreviations: HIPAA, Health Insurance Portability and Accountability Act; LIS, laboratory information system; RFP, request for proposal.
Adapted from Henricks WH, Boyer PJ, Harrison JH, et al. Informatics training in pathology residency programs: proposed learning objectives and skill sets for the new millennium. Arch Pathol Lab Med 2003;127:1009–18.

surgical pathology through both real time and historical cases; this same pattern adapts well to the learning PI.

The doing component of learning that fully demonstrates competency is never fully accomplished by didactic methods, updating a wiki, discussing a business-style case study, and/or self-paced learning from a textbook or virtual rotation. The authors have observed, however, that resident engagement in longitudinal projects seems highly valuable in cementing the skills needed to achieve the level of performance competency required. **Table 4** lists a sampling of resident-led longitudinal learning projects, some of which resulted in publications; many of these have significant informatics components. These kinds of doing projects, however, seldom fit nicely into a 2- to 4-week elective, or informatics block, in the resident schedule. So how do programs and learners find the time to allow this kind of experience when so much of their other clinical material–based learning is neatly divided into time-based blocks? Different

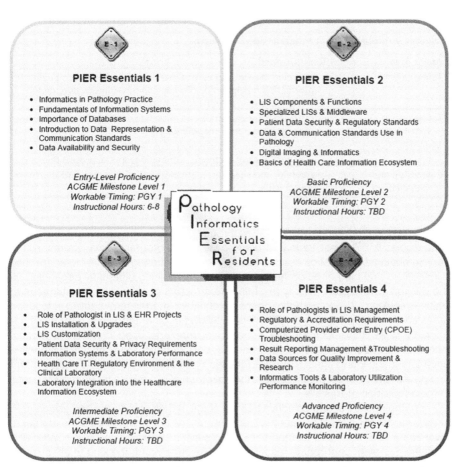

PIER Essentials 1

- Informatics in Pathology Practice
- Fundamentals of Information Systems
- Importance of Databases
- Introduction to Data Representation & Communication Standards
- Data Availability and Security

Entry-Level Proficiency
ACGME Milestone Level 1
Workable Timing: PGY 1
Instructional Hours: 6-8

PIER Essentials 2

- LIS Components & Functions
- Specialized LISs & Middleware
- Patient Data Security & Regulatory Standards
- Data & Communication Standards Use in Pathology
- Digital Imaging & Informatics
- Basics of Health Care Information Ecosystem

Basic Proficiency
ACGME Milestone Level 2
Workable Timing: PGY 2
Instructional Hours: TBD

Pathology Informatics Essentials for Residents

PIER Essentials 3

- Role of Pathologist in LIS & EHR Projects
- LIS Installation & Upgrades
- LIS Customization
- Patient Data Security & Privacy Requirements
- Information Systems & Laboratory Performance
- Health Care IT Regulatory Environment & the Clinical Laboratory
- Laboratory Integration into the Healthcare Information Ecosystem

Intermediate Proficiency
ACGME Milestone Level 3
Workable Timing: PGY 3
Instructional Hours: TBD

PIER Essentials 4

- Role of Pathologists in LIS Management
- Regulatory & Accreditation Requirements
- Computerized Provider Order Entry (CPOE) Troubleshooting
- Result Reporting Management & Troubleshooting
- Data Sources for Quality Improvement & Research
- Informatics Tools & Laboratory Utilization /Performance Monitoring

Advanced Proficiency
ACGME Milestone Level 4
Workable Timing: PGY 4
Instructional Hours: TBD

Fig. 1. Informatics core curriculum for residency training as proposed by API, APC, and CAP to meet Milestone SBP7. EHR, electronic health record; PGY, post-graduate year; TBD, to be determined. (*From* Association of Pathology Chairs. Pathology Informatics Essentials for Residents instructional resource guide. Available at: http://www.apcprods.org/pier/documents/PIERIRG_Release0_July2014_v1.pdf; with permission).

programs use different strategies to accomplish this, although informal surveys indicate that few programs require or significantly (ie, structurally) facilitate these kinds of hands-on resident projects. At the University of Oklahoma, such projects typically occur during a senior integrated rotation covering 3 months, during which they assume a variety of high-level duties. This timing, however, often does not allow the luxury of seeing the follow-up stage of project implementation. To counter this problem, programs may pair residents of different years. Another program has proposed chartering long-term projects early in training and using a time bank of resident elective time to offer short-term coverage for needed activities when a resident is engaged in a clinically demanding rotation (Massachusetts General Hospital forum on clinical informatics, 2014, personal communication).

Fellowship-level training in PI pertinent to surgical/anatomic pathology builds on the resident experience foundation that has been developed. Several models have been used, but many seem to draw on the diversity of individual fellow experiences to enrich

Table 3	
Didactic curriculum content for postresidency training	
Major Area	Topics Covered
Information	Information theory, information architecture, information quality, information manipulation, human-computer interaction, design principles, special information domains
Information systems	Infrastructure fundamentals, LIS, interfaces, system life cycle, health information systems, imaging systems
Workflow and process	Process and quality improvement, business process management, workflow analysis methods, automation, special process domains
Leadership and management	Leadership, management, regulation, teams, cross-organizational project issues

the whole, contemporaneously as well as through revival of prior projects in the form of case studies.[9,15,16] These various structured fellowship programs have addressed the varying anticipated practice needs of their fellows by offering flexibility to adapt their experiences and the period or duration of fellowship training differently depending on the desired career path. This type of flexible structuring, although advantageous to trainees seeking a broad portfolio, opens potential for shorter-term training in focused areas and may help existing practitioners or fellows in other pathology disciplines acquire PI skills.[16] Additionally, the educational methods used in these programs, including operational projects, research time, core didactic sessions, clinical conference attendance, and special retreats focused on decision-making and management and governance issues, nicely capture the spectrum of modalities thought most useful in the acquisition of PI skills.

For pathologists beyond an active training stage of their career, the acquisition of PI skills is harder to gauge for a variety of reasons. On the one hand, need is the mother of invention and a motivated learner, seeking to solve a vexing problem, is a more efficient learner given appropriate resources. On the other hand, the kind of effective instruction that may make this learning less painful is often not available for subject matter like PI. Consultation on mobile surgical pathology materials is simple to obtain, even from experts in another country. But finding the right consultant/teacher for a longer-term informatics problem is harder, given (1) the limited number of known well-trained practitioners and (2) the lack of a readily available reimbursement structure to gain access to or interest from the consultant/teacher. National meetings of pathology-related organizations often include informatics topics, although some attendees have contended that the relative quantity of programs has diminished over the past decade whereas the need has been increasing. Several excellent textbooks covering the full range of PI have been published, partially filling the IT learning gaps as far as the foundational core is concerned, but these tend to offer little when it comes to solving a particular IT problem.

Box 1
Keys to making pathology informatics work in residency training
Engage learners to master core content, such as through a wiki.
Provide regular exposure to diverse live and historical informatics case examples.
Promote participation in longitudinal projects requiring application of PI skills.

Table 4
Sample resident informatics projects

Project Synopsis	Estimated Time Frame	Comments
Closing the loop with critical action results—project to ensure that significant LIS-generated results triggered EMR response, including follow-up visit scheduling and/or risk management notice	3–6 mo	The number of stakeholders, critical partners, or institutions involved tends to multiply the time required
Standardizing evidence-based care and appropriate utilization of esoteric hematopathology testing—project involving redesign of ordering tools and processes to optimize specimen procurement and test ordering, applying decision-support tools at the appropriate stage	9 mo (multiple iterations required)	Savings provided to institution and payers helped support further projects
Implementation of a decision support tool to optimize IHC utilization	3 mo	Accrued benefits to health system required 6 mo to 1 y to measure meaningfully
Revision of processes and tools for enhanced accuracy of surgical case coding	2–4 mo	

LABORATORY INFORMATICS TRAINING AT THE UNIVERSITY OF OKLAHOMA

The authors' informatics core rotation consists of 14 1-week blocks (as shown in **Table 5**). In block A, initial lectures focus on laboratory information systems (LIS) and include an overview of the different areas of computerization required for modern laboratory practice: LIS for the clinical laboratory, LIS for the anatomic pathology laboratory, laboratory billing systems, and office automation computing and networking. Possible stand-alone subsystem computers for more specialized laboratory sections are also discussed, which may include Food and Drug Administration–approved transfusion medicine applications, molecular pathology systems, so-called big data–associated applications, middleware for point-of-care testing outreach program, and middleware for total track automation systems in the core clinical laboratory. These preliminary lectures include the types of computer hardware and software required for the various topographies of systems available: (1) local area networks deploying intelligent client workstations, (2) central mainframe computers deploying intelligent workstations running emulation software, and (3) central mainframe computers using a central core database deploying essential thin clients with so-called dumb workstations. A discussion is included of the type of equipment required in the traditional laboratory computer center, the specialized ambient environmental and security requirements, fire protections, system backup devices and media and media security/storage, daily central computer maintenance and management requirements, system updates including procedures for tracking new versions and changes, maintaining a test environment for evaluation/testing of new or modified applications prior to implementation on the live system, and disk maintenance routines including compression and elimination of disk fragments. It is stressed that (1) the continuous availability of all computer systems is essential for the operation of the

Table 5
Organization of core lectures in laboratory informatics at University of Oklahoma pathology training program—1 week per block

Block A	Introduction to laboratory computers Clinical laboratory computerization Anatomic pathology computerization Business computing Office computing and networking
Block B	Use of computers in laboratory statistics Statistics of quality control Statistical tests of significance
Block C	Use of spreadsheets for statistics MediCalc and other statistics programs Receiver operator curves Integration of graphs with laboratory statistics
Block D	Bits and bytes Programming a laboratory computer Operating system/system tools Job control languages, scripts Application programming Screens, navigation tools, graphic user interfaces
Block E	Database concepts/file design PC database tools for design, creation, and maintenance Requisite files in APLIS Query tools, sorting, control breaks, record selection criteria Reporting tools and graphics
Block F	Selection of an LIS/replacement of LIS Implementation issues Connectivity and interfaces Backup and maintenance System support and data recovery issues Security, firewalls, HIPAA requirements
Block G	Operation of an LIS Required functionality and programs Core clinical laboratory computerization Point-of-care testing computerization Blood bank system Microbiology system AP system
Block H	Business computing Coding, billing, and compliance issues Web-based computing Process/project management and simulation tools
Block I	Presentation tools PowerPoint and other presentation software Animation tools Multimedia and PowerPoint Digital presentation issues
Block J	Imaging and computerization Image capture, slide scanning, digital photography Merging images and text in presentations Image storage Voice recognition

(continued on next page)

Table 5 (continued)	
Block K	Office automation Word processing tools Scheduling and time management tools E-mail Mobile computing—PDAs, laptops, other mobile devices
Block L	Internet or Web-based activity in the laboratory or clinic Creating and maintaining a Web site Medical reporting using online submission Internet search for educational materials Citation management software
Block M	Laboratory computer standards—ASTM, HL7, LOINC, CIC Interfacing of laboratory equipment Total laboratory automation and connectivity issues EDI (?) interfacing vs scripted approach Scripting and emulation tools Web portals for order entry and results reporting
Block N	LIS management issues Software and hardware support, internal and external Personnel issues—training and competency Table and file maintenance Clinical issues and system requirements Paperless printing and electronic reporting Expert systems and decision support; evidence-based medicine support

Abbreviations: ASTM, American Society for Testing Materials; CIC, connectivity industry consortium; EDI, electronic data interchange; HL7, health level 7; LOINC, logical observation identifiers names and codes.

laboratory and (2) a knowledgeable well-trained pathologist in IT has the overall responsibility of maintaining the full function, reliability, and security of all IT systems critical to the patient care mission of the laboratory.

The various staffing requirements of the LIS section as part of block A are discussed, including (1) laboratory data center managers, (2) database specialists, (3) system programmers, (4) system security officer, and (5) system operations personnel. Requirements for bench-level computer experts in each laboratory section are also focused on, with technologists assigned responsibility for (1) operation systems software on laboratory instruments and associated interface software; (2) middleware software for system monitoring, interfacing, and autovalidation; and (3) tracking automation software and associated interfaces and networking. Personnel required for laboratory billing applications are discussed as well, including (1) charge capture and coding personnel; (2) accounts receivable and payments posting; (3) audits for billing compliance and accounting purposes and associated accounts management; (4) billing statements, cycles, reporting, delinquent accounts, and collections referrals; and (5) billing compliance personnel. Also, paperless middleware support for ongoing documentation of CLIA'88, the Joint Commission, and CAP compliance is essential for efficient laboratory practice and accreditation. Staffing for this application must be considered as part of a laboratory IT team.

During the first blocks, the rotation focuses on the so-called language of computers, which begin with the basis of computer operation at the bit and byte levels and then progresses to terms essential for describing and understanding the disk operating system software, associated hardware, computer memory, binary coding systems for numbers and text, and the unique nature of different types of data (numerical, text, alphanumeric, floating point data, integers, coded hex, ASCII codes, binary vs decimal, and conversions), documents, images, and space requirements for data storage in memory and disk storage. Computer programming languages are described along with concepts of compilers, job control language, scripting languages, macros, and interpretive computer languages. Early sessions (block D) include exercises in software development using off-the-shelf tools and freeware, such as the Basic computer language. Each resident is required to develop and test at least 5 different programs, with each project solving specific laboratory-based problems. These exercises include the use of programming approaches to use for (1) decision loops, (2) user-interactive screen prompts, (3) calculations using structured language approaches, (4) variable types including subscripted variables and arrays, (5) subroutines and branching, and (6) results output displays and printing including formatting with captions and headings. The authors' experience with the programming exercises suggests that these exercises facilitate a better understanding of how computers actually work in terms of hardware, terms, and functions. They also assist pathology residents' understanding of the limitations of various computer functions and tools.

For interactive programming, screen design programming tools are also discussed as part of block D. Graphic interface tools are included in this section and include concepts of program calls with command lines, program menu screens, and graphic user interface icons/object–oriented approaches. Keyboard tools and mouse functions are included in this discussion as well. After discussions and exercises covered in blocks A through D, the residents are assigned security passwords with more capability and permissions, which allow them to be trained more thoroughly on the LIS systems.

Blocks E and F focus on issues that must be considered prior to the acquisition of an LIS. These blocks include concepts of file design with a focus on tools that allow access into various data elements stored therein. Structured query tools are covered along with exercises to create databases that can be sorted, searched, and processed. These topics include data extraction along with migration of data into various PC-based applications, including spreadsheets and local databases. Record layouts with various file organization, including sequential and indexed files, are covered. Various types of data fields for laboratory applications are discussed, along with the required characteristics of various data fields in databases, in these blocks. Boolean logic and decision support concepts are included in these blocks, with specific examples of structured query approaches using the appropriate data extraction and processing logic. System selection and system replacement criteria are included with emphasis on project risk, especially those risks pertaining to uncontrollable project variables, which may include system interfacing, overall system reliability, total system costs, and system capacity/speed.

Blocks G though K of the Oklahoma resident IT training program focus mostly on the day-to-day operational aspects of the LIS (see **Table 5**). These sessions drill down into the details of the operation of each type of LIS used in the laboratory, with emphasis on the unique role of each LIS system deployed. These blocks also include more detail on the power of the individual workstations and deployed emulation software thereon. Some of these workstation tools have very useful capability, including scripting tools for specialized applications.

Block L focuses on Web-based programming and applications on mobile devices, including a discussion of Java programming and cloud-based computing. Various devices can be used in this block for exercises, including Android smartphones and tablets. Laboratory interface standards are covered in block M: American Society for

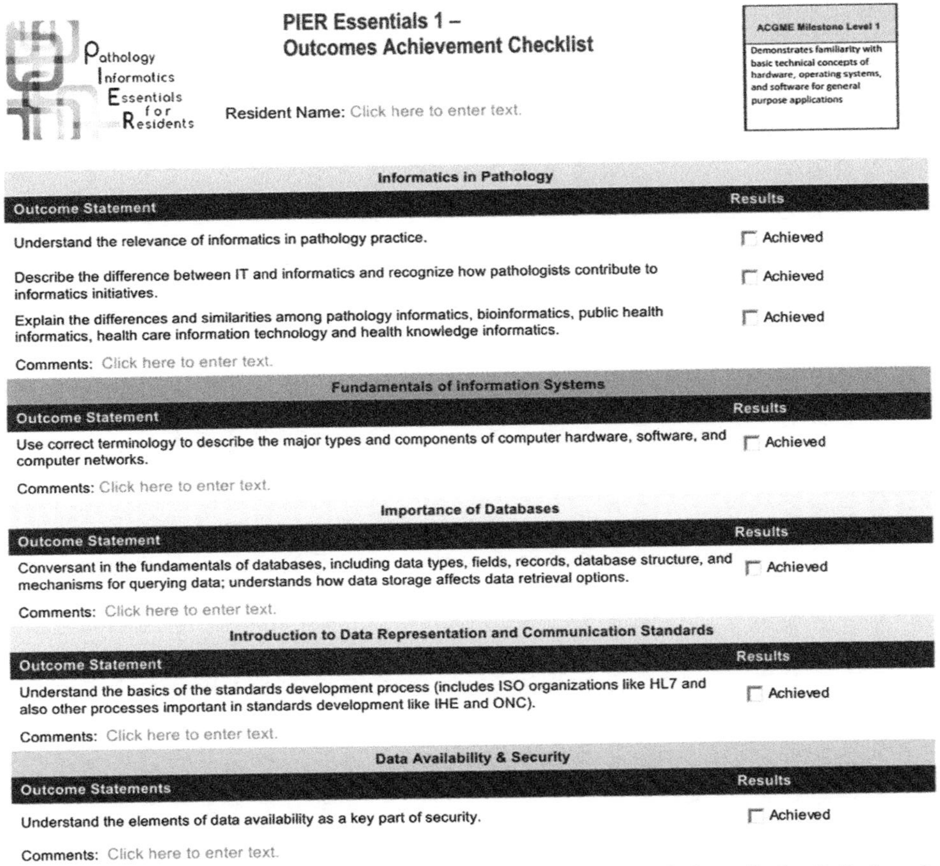

PIER Essentials 1 –
Outcomes Achievement Checklist

Pathology
Informatics
Essentials
for
Residents

Resident Name: Click here to enter text.

ACGME Milestone Level 1
Demonstrates familiarity with basic technical concepts of hardware, operating systems, and software for general purpose applications

Informatics in Pathology

Outcome Statement	Results
Understand the relevance of informatics in pathology practice.	⊓ Achieved
Describe the difference between IT and informatics and recognize how pathologists contribute to informatics initiatives.	⊓ Achieved
Explain the differences and similarities among pathology informatics, bioinformatics, public health informatics, health care information technology and health knowledge informatics.	⊓ Achieved

Comments: Click here to enter text.

Fundamentals of Information Systems

Outcome Statement	Results
Use correct terminology to describe the major types and components of computer hardware, software, and computer networks.	⊓ Achieved

Comments: Click here to enter text.

Importance of Databases

Outcome Statement	Results
Conversant in the fundamentals of databases, including data types, fields, records, database structure, and mechanisms for querying data; understands how data storage affects data retrieval options.	⊓ Achieved

Comments: Click here to enter text.

Introduction to Data Representation and Communication Standards

Outcome Statement	Results
Understand the basics of the standards development process (includes ISO organizations like HL7 and also other processes important in standards development like IHE and ONC).	⊓ Achieved

Comments: Click here to enter text.

Data Availability & Security

Outcome Statements	Results
Understand the elements of data availability as a key part of security.	⊓ Achieved

Comments: Click here to enter text.

Fig. 2. PIER outcomes achievement checklist tool for documentation. (*From* Association of Pathology Chairs. Pathology Informatics Essentials for Residents instructional resource guide. Available at: http://www.apcprods.org/pier/documents/PIERIRG_Release0_July2014_v1.pdf; with permission.)

Testing Materials (ASTM) and Health Level Seven International (HL7) standards for data interchange between instruments and the LIS. Interfacing between hospital information systems and electronic medical records (EMR) systems and LIS systems using the HL7 standards are also covered. The final block, block N, of the rotation reviews the main points covered in the entire resident IT program, again with an emphasis on daily operations and system reliability issues. The focus is on the overall responsibility of IT-trained pathologists in the success of a laboratory, which, going forward, is largely determined by the success of the IT deployment and day-to-day operations.

Long-term resident project conceptualization, development, implementation, and monitoring have yet to be entirely successfully structured into the program for every resident, although there have been several individual successes on these components of training, such as those listed in **Table 4**. The model covers the core content well but is faculty intensive. Resources, such as those newly assembled and packaged by API, CAP, and APC as the PIER resource guide, seem to make the acquisition of the core didactic content more readily available to more residents[17] and to facilitate documentation of progress (**Fig. 2**).

SUMMARY

This article presents an overview and considerable detail of the curriculum that the authors and others deem essential for trainees in pathology. These are closely tied to the competencies desired for pathology graduates and ultimately practitioners. The value of case (problem)-based learning in this realm is emphasized, in particular the kind of integrative experience associated with hands-on projects, to cement knowledge gained in the lecture hall or online and to expand competency.

REFERENCES

1. Naritoku WY, Alexander CB, Bennett BD, et al. The pathology milestones and the next accreditation system. Arch Pathol Lab Med 2014;138:307–15.
2. Nasca TJ, Philibert I, Brigham T, et al. The next GME accreditation system—rationale and benefits. N Engl J Med 2012;366:1051–6.
3. Swing SR, Clyman SG, Holmboe ES, et al. Advancing resident assessment in graduate medical education. J Grad Med Educ 2009;1:278–86.
4. Henricks WH, Boyer PJ, Harrison JH, et al. Informatics training in pathology residency programs: proposed learning objectives and skill sets for the new millennium. Arch Pathol Lab Med 2003;127:1009–18.
5. The pathology milestone project. J Grad Med Educ 2014;4:183.
6. Tischler AS. Pheochromocytoma: time to stamp out "malignancy"? Endocr Pathol 2008;19:207–8.
7. Gabril MY, Yousef GM. Informatics for practicing anatomical pathologists: marking a new era in pathology practice. Mod Pathol 2010;23:349–58.
8. Gilbertson JR, McClintock DS, Lee RE, et al. Clinical fellowship training in pathology informatics: a program description. J Pathol Inform 2012;3:11.
9. Pantanowitz L, Tuthill JM, Balis UG, editors. Pathology informatics: theory and practice. Chicago, IL: ASCP Press; 2012.
10. Sinard J. Practical pathology informatics: demystifying informatics for the practicing anatomic pathologist. New York, NY: Springer; 2006.
11. Park S, Parwani A, MacPherson T, et al. Use of a wiki as an interactive teaching tool in pathology residency education: Experience with a genomics, research, and informatics in pathology course. J Pathol Inform 2012;3:32.

12. Kang HP, Hagenkord JM, Monzon FA, et al. Residency Training in Pathology Informatics A Virtual Rotation Solution. Am J Clin Pathol 2009;132:404–8.
13. Kohli MD, Bradshaw JK. What is a wiki, and how can it be used in resident education? J Digit Imaging 2011;24:170–5.
14. ASCP/APF, Lab Management University. Available at: http://www.ascp.org/PDF/LMU/FAQs-v4.pdf. Accessed August 6, 2014.
15. Quinn A, Klepeis V, Mandelker D, et al. The ongoing evolution of the core curriculum of a clinical fellowship in pathology informatics. J Pathol Inform 2014;5:22.
16. Levy BP, McClintock DS, Lee RE, et al. Different tracks for pathology informatics fellowship training: Experiences of and input from trainees in a large multisite fellowship program. J Pathol Inform 2012;3:30.
17. Henricks W, Pantanowitz L, Powell SZ, et al. PIER Instructional Resource Guide. 2014. Available at: http://www.apcprods.org/pier/documents/PIERIRG_Release0_July2014_v1.pdf. Accessed August 18, 2014.

Printed and bound by CPI Group (UK) Ltd, Croydon, CR0 4YY

07/10/2024

01040505-0018